Eat, Drink, and Be Wary

Praise for *Eat, Drink, and Be Wary*

"*Eat, Drink, and Be Wary* comes as a rude awakening to the fact that our government is asleep at the wheel in safeguarding our foods. In this book, Charles M. Duncan has reminded us about the horrifying truth of the deteriorating quality of foods we consume daily. He also informs us, the consumers, as to what we can do to reverse this destructive trend." —**Chensheng Alex Lu**, PhD, associate professor of environmental exposure biology, Harvard School of Public Health

"In *Eat, Drink, and Be Wary* Duncan offers us a gruesome panorama of the global food industry, its frailties and its dangers. If we considered food to be a more critical factor in health, we might inspect and care for this system differently. But as Duncan shows, food is but a commodity, inspected and monitored by a lackadaisical political system, created and sold at minimal cost to consumers who are anonymous and replaceable. This book is a quick overview, product by product, crisis by crisis, of the current dangers in our industrial foods." —**Carolyn Smith-Morris**, PhD, MS, LPC, associate professor, Southern Methodist University

"A great repository of facts for anyone who is concerned about food safety. It is a much needed outcry for transparency in our food production." —**Mark Post**, MD, PhD, professor and chair of physiology, Maastricht University

"Foodborne illnesses and the quality of food production and preparation are major issues in the United States. This is a must-read for every parent and for anyone interested in their general health. The more knowledgeable we are the more transparent and accountable the industry must become. The quality of our food should always be held to the highest standards and not allowed to continue to be a form of culinary Russian roulette." —**Bill Macatee**, announcer for the NFL on CBS, US Open Tennis, golf

"In his carefully researched book, Charles M. Duncan comprehensively addresses hazards as they come with our daily food. Based on solid facts, figures, and references, he fascinatingly discusses nutritional safety and security across the board: from bioterrorism over food imports and genetically modified organisms to outbreaks of foodborne illnesses, and others. The book also includes honed criticism of the dispersion of responsibility in the U.S. system of government, as well as practical tips on how to mitigate food-related risks in our everyday lives. This work is an excellent contribution to fostering homeland and civil security debates in an all-hazards context, as well as to increasing societal awareness and preparedness." —**Alexander Siedschlag**, PhD, professor and chair of Homeland Security and Public Health Preparedness, The Pennsylvania State University, Penn State Harrisburg

"For Americans, eating healthy may only be a challenge at the start of our daily routine. Finding a variety of safe, healthy, and available foods impacts the health of us all. As some of our everyday interactions have been marked with more invasiveness, Duncan poses questions on food safety, trends in risk management with nutrition, and concerns with the oversight needed to prevent food threats from natural hazards to terrorism. Information on eating safely may be a new top of the food pyramid." —**J. Eric Dietz**, PhD, PE, director, Purdue Homeland Security Institute, and professor of computer and information technology

"Charles Duncan has provided a sobering, and potentially stomach-churning, look at the gaps in our food safety system. Controls on food imports are negligible, domestic controls are too lax, and food producers are taking short-cuts and risks that should alarm every consumer." —**Wayne Pacelle**, president and CEO, The Humane Society of the United States

"A must-read for policy makers and elected officials—while they are eating! Duncan documents one of the most important crises in America—the safety of our food." —**David A. Sterling**, PhD, CIH, professor and chair of the Department of Environmental and Occupational Health Sciences, director doctoral PhD program, School of Public Health, University of North Texas Health Science Center

"A lot of the information Charles Duncan includes in *Eat, Drink, and Be Wary*, is scary as hell! However, by reading this book, we will all be better informed about the choices we make and the foods we eat. Thank you Charles and BON APPETIT ya'll!" —**Ruta Lee**, Canadian actress, Hollywood, California

"Charles M. Duncan has assembled a significant amount of data on the problems with allowing uninspected and untested food products to enter the marketplace. Duncan outlines the major failures of the government agencies in allowing healthy food to reach the tabletop." —**John Ubelaker**, PhD, Southern Methodist University

"*Eat, Drink, and Be Wary* is a detailed examination of the failure of government oversight agencies to protect consumers from food companies that place profit above everything else. This failure of the agencies that are supposed to oversee the food industries leads to horrible cruelty to farm animals and a polluted food supply. You will cry and, if you have a dark sense of humor, you will laugh. My hope is that you will also be spurred to action." —**Bruce Friedrich**, director of advocacy and policy, Farm Sanctuary

Eat, Drink, and Be Wary

How Unsafe Is Our Food?

Charles M. Duncan

EDITED BY DIANA KEARLEY DUNCAN

ROWMAN & LITTLEFIELD
Lanham • Boulder • New York • London

Published by Rowman & Littlefield
A wholly owned subsidiary of The Rowman & Littlefield Publishing Group, Inc.
4501 Forbes Boulevard, Suite 200, Lanham, Maryland 20706
www.rowman.com

Unit A, Whitacre Mews, 26-34 Stannary Street, London SE11 4AB

British Library Cataloguing in Publication Information Available

Library of Congress Cataloging-in-Publication Data

Duncan, Charles, author.
Eat, drink, and be wary : how unsafe is our food? / Charles M. Duncan.
p. ; cm.
Includes bibliographical references and index.
ISBN 978-1-4422-3839-8 (cloth : alk. paper) -- ISBN 978-1-4422-3840-4 (electronic)
I. Title.
DNLM: 1. Food Safety -- United States. 2. Bioterrorism -- United States. 3. Drug Resistance, Bacterial -- United States. 4. Food Contamination -- United States. 5. Foodborne Diseases -- United States. WA 695].
RA601.5 2015
363.19'26--dc23
2014026995

♾ ™ The paper used in this publication meets the minimum requirements of American National Standard for Information Sciences Permanence of Paper for Printed Library Materials, ANSI/NISO Z39.48-1992.

Printed in the United States of America

I dedicate this book to my untiring wife, Diana Kearley Duncan, who persistently spent untold hours proofing and editing *Eat, Drink, and Be Wary: How Unsafe Is Our Food?* Diana helped research many areas of food safety and gave me encouragement and the momentum to keep up a sometimes-frantic pace. She unselfishly put on hold a book she was starting to write in order to lend her support to this project in numerous ways.

Dedicating *Eat, Drink, and Be Wary* to Diana is accompanied by my overwhelming love and joy to be with this hugely successful business-woman, a dear and dedicated friend to many and a loving wife to me.

Contents

Foreword

Following the shocking disclosures of unsanitary conditions in American meat-packing plants, the Federal Meat Inspection Act and the Pure Food and Drugs Act were passed by Congress on June 30, 1906. They were signed into law by President Theodore Roosevelt, who had been disgusted by the slaughterhouse practices described in Upton Sinclair's book, *The Jungle*. These Acts provided for the federal regulation of meat, poultry, and egg products and prohibited the interstate commerce of misbranded and adulterated foods and drinks. Today, there are 15 federal agencies, including the Food and Drug Administration, implementing at least 30 laws related to food safety. However, even with these agencies and laws to protect us, thousands die, hundreds of thousands are hospitalized and millions are sickened by the food they eat. Almost daily in the media and on the internet we read or see stories of those affected. And almost every one of us has experienced food poisoning resulting from eating out or even from food prepared in our own kitchen. Unfortunately, this highly significant public health problem has motivated too little public outcry and has resulted in minimal action on behalf of citizens by our local, state and federal legislators.

In *Eat, Drink, and Be Wary: How Unsafe Is Our Food?* Charles M. Duncan has compiled a cross-sectional analysis of every aspect of the food industry, with crucial safety ramifications that can impact all of us. I first met Charles Duncan when he was an investigative reporter with KAKE-TV in Wichita Kansas. At that time I was the director of the Wichita–Sedgwick County Department of Community Health. The station had been running an investigative series featuring Charles, called "Let's Eat Out," which was examining unsanitary conditions in some of Wichita's restaurants. The station advocated for a restaurant rating system which I also supported and subsequently put in place.

Eat, Drink, and Be Wary: How Unsafe Is Our Food? delves into the problems we as consumers face regarding nearly everything we eat everyday—produce, poultry, meat products, seafood, dairy—and reveals how poorly our government, at all levels, protects us. The information that Charles Duncan has gathered for this book may be sufficient to have all of us fantasizing a return to a time when families lived more basically, raising animals and growing produce for their own sustenance. Not only are the goods provided us from our own producers untrustworthy, but the commodities we import, and which make up over 10 percent of our diet, undergo virtually no inspection. To add insult to injury, a number of countries—some with the worst records of contaminated food exports—prohibit the importing of genetically modified foods, and foods containing harmful additives and/or bacteria, from the United States! And who can blame them? All of the countries of the European Union and many other nations around the world, using the same data available to us, have much stricter guidelines on food additives than we do. What do they know that we don't?

Our federal governmental agencies seem to have lost their way when it comes to acting in accordance with the original language of the Federal Food and Drugs Act of 1906, which was designed to safeguard us. The infrequency of inspections, the seeming collusion between the regulators and the regulated, and the insufficient funding for agencies established to protect the supply, processing, importation and sale of foods, leaves the American consumer seriously vulnerable. When we consider such dangerous practices as the extensive use of antibiotics and harmful additives, the contamination of food products due to carelessness during growth and preparation for market, and the purposeful mislabeling of products, we recognize just how far we have strayed from the intent of the Federal Food and Drugs Act. People who resent paying taxes for government oversight or who oppose regulation in principle, might want to reconsider. If they are not concerned about the welfare of the public at large, they might at least want to become informed as to what is in their own self-interest.

Charles could have entitled his book, "Let the Buyer Beware," and certainly a careful reading will make the buyer beware. Hopefully there will be a groundswell of public demand for a food industry that is safe and responsive to the needs of the consuming public. *Eat, Drink, and Be Wary: How Unsafe Is Our Food?* is a wake-up call. We can continue to ignore what exists, or, using this book as an important resource, we can question our food suppliers about their sources and practices, and contact the relevant agencies whenever we observe a food-borne issue. Beyond this, we must be willing to voice our desire for greater regulation and to pressure our elected officials. They need our strong support so that they can succeed in enacting legislation to provide adequate funding and effective enforcement of measures that will ensure food safety for us all. Charles Duncan has taken a major step in doing the comprehensive research and writing this important book. The rest is up to us.

Mervyn F. Silverman, M.D., M.P.H.

Former director of the Office of Consumer Affairs, FDA

Former director of the Wichita–Sedgwick County Department of Community Health, Wichita Kansas

Former director of Health for the City and County of San Francisco, California

Acknowledgments

So many people have contributed so much throughout my journalism career, leading me to this most exciting and gratifying moment—writing *Eat, Drink, and Be Wary: How Unsafe Is Our Food?* Here are just a few of the terrific people who have inspired and helped along the way:

Nelson Galle and J. K. Lane gave me major responsibilities at KHBR Radio in Hillsboro, Texas, even before I graduated from high school. They gave me the confidence and encouragement that quickly moved me along in my broadcast journalism career.

Martin Umansky, a graduate of the highly regarded University of Missouri School of Journalism. He was president and owner of KAKE-TV in Wichita, Kansas, but journalism always came first. Martin's dedication to the First Amendment and the public's right to know had its price tag in major losses of advertisers who disagreed with our social discrimination investigations and our straightforward facts about filthy, roach-infested restaurants.

Larry Hatteberg, who has worked for about 50 years at KAKE-TV in Wichita, Kansas, as chief photographer, news director, and anchor. He was National News Photographer of the Year for several years. Thanks to Larry for the many valuable on-the-scene lessons in photojournalism he provided me.

Tracy Rowlett, long-time news anchor and award-winning reporter at WFAA-TV in Dallas, who helped me move up from a terrific position in the news department at KAKE-TV in Wichita to the even more prestigious and progressive newsroom of WFAA-TV in Dallas, known nationally as one of the best in the nation at the time.

Marty Haag, news director at WFAA-TV in Dallas and later the Vice President for News for Belo television stations nationwide. Marty allowed me the necessary time and travel to thoroughly research and produce news documentaries and investigative series. He encouraged me to expand my *Eat, Drink, and Be Wary* series of critical food safety problems in restaurants to include all phases of food issues.

Doug Fox and John Sparks, award-winning reporter and producer, respectively, who wielded a mean red pen when editing my rough drafts.

Former lawmen and undercover agents Gary Howard and Ron Tucker, who trusted me enough to bring me into an 18-month-long top secret federal undercover U.S. Customs and ATF sting operation, targeting one of the world's most ruthless international arms dealers. Britain's Ian Smalley armed both sides of the 1980s Iran-Iraq war with illegal sales of tanks, missiles, and ammunition.

Ed Bark, nationally known former Dallas Morning News TV and radio critic, past president of the Television Critics Association, and a seven-year member of the national Peabody Awards board. Ed never minded stepping on a few toes and kept most of the reporters on their toes as he constantly looked over our shoulders. Still doing the same at http//www.unclebarky.com.

Kassie Wegner, Daniel Lewandowski, and all the extremely helpful, friendly, and professional people at the Alfred C. O'Connell Library at Genesee Community College in Batavia, New York, I thank you.

Richardson, Texas, Public Library staff, my thanks to all of you.

Introduction

Eat, Drink, and Be Wary describes our enormous food safety problems, the vast scope of each dangerous issue, the many reasons why our government can't get a grip on these escalating and potentially deadly problems, and our lax efforts in an all-out attack on our deteriorating state of food safety.

In the United States, foodborne illness deaths number more than 3,000 each year; 128,000 are hospitalized from such illness; and foodborne sicknesses hit 48 million others. Although the response from the U.S. Food and Drug Administration (FDA) in April 2014 was, "This is a significant public health burden that is largely preventable," there's no evidence of a move toward prevention. The FDA:

- inspects less than 2 percent of the 10 million food shipments arriving each year at our ports;
- fails to inspect 90 percent of the potentially deadly high-priority overseas food sources, including China, Korea, and India, as required;
- cuts back the number of inspectors at key food processing locations and orders less time be spent physically examining poultry;
- favors the big food-manufacturing giants on enforcement issues while it should be protecting consumers and the food we eat; and
- allows food manufacturers to make their own determination as to the safety of chemicals and food additives.

You will see throughout this book how our government fails in its responsibilities to "protect the public health by assuring that foods are safe, wholesome, sanitary, and properly labeled." The staggering number of Americans who get sick or die from food is indicative of the alarming state of our food safety and sends out calls for a transfusion of changes, if not flatline resuscitation. The statistics repeat annually.

Our food safety levels began faltering around 2005. The following years saw major outbreaks of foodborne diseases coupled with massive recalls of lettuce, spinach, and peanut butter. The illnesses and deaths increased.

I address every food group and its potential dangers in *Eat, Drink, and Be Wary: How Unsafe Is Our Food?* Foodborne illnesses strike one out of six people in the United States each year. Contaminations permeate each phase of our food chain, from the wheat and corn fields, grazing cattle, slaughterhouses, egg farms, and dairies to our oceans and bays, and on the loading docks and airports where imports arrive from around the world. Potential poisons lurk at every stop along the way to our kitchens and restaurants. The culprits include pesticides, arsenic, Salmonella, E. coli, Botulinum, and Listeria coupled with lax laws, few inspections, and poor enforcement. Potential bioterrorism and cyber attacks directed at our food and water supplies pose another major danger facing this country's effort to protect the food we eat.

The bureaucracy within U.S. food safety agencies over the years escalated to a contest, bigger than the Super Bowl, between the FDA and the USDA (U.S. Department of Agriculture), a race for more dominance, power, and control. Enforcement of convoluted regulations often favors giant food corporations while ignoring the health and safety of consumers.

Numerous surveys of Americans vividly demonstrate the concerns most consumers have about our food safety. Nearly three-quarters of Americans want more government oversight in food safety. A February 2014 Harris poll of 2,236 adults reveals that food recalls have consumers at least somewhat concerned or seriously concerned.[1] Over half (86 percent) of the U.S. adults in the survey indicated that if a brand they usually purchase became involved with a recall or safety concern issue, they would temporarily switch to another brand.

Hopefully you will find that the following chapters address your questions, concerns, and worries about our food. I have also compiled a list of expert sources (see the appendix) you may contact for further information about pathogens, outbreaks, and other food safety issues.

Chapter One

Bioterrorism, Cyber Attacks

"It is highly unlikely that acts of food terrorism can be completely prevented." This is a straightforward warning from the respected World Health Organization (WHO).[1] "Food is the most vulnerable to intentional contamination by debilitating or lethal agents. The diversity of sources of foods, including the global market, makes prevention difficult."

The media reported dire warnings as far back as 2003: "Terrorists can produce Salmonella and Botulinum with an aim at poisoning troops in Afghanistan," wrote Barton Gellman in the *Washington Post*.[2]

U.S. troops entered the caves and safe houses of members of the Al Qaeda terrorist network in Afghanistan in the months following the September 11 attacks. Hundreds of pages of U.S. agriculture documents translated into Arabic had been left behind. Troops discovered a significant part of the group's training manual devoted to agricultural terrorism—specifically, the destruction of crops, livestock, and food processing operations.

Katherine McIntire Peters, writing for the Government Executive website, said, "Many agricultural experts believe the greatest threat to U.S. agriculture would be the deliberate or accidental introduction of foot-and-mouth disease, the highly contagious viral disease that attacks cloven-footed animals, including cattle, swine, sheep, deer and elk."[3] While humans cannot contract the disease from animals, its effect on animals is so swift and debilitating that milk and meat production could be severely cut nationwide. With thousands of animals being transported across state lines every week, "an outbreak could spread within days, before animal health officials could provide a definitive diagnosis," she wrote.

Peters also pointed out that even rumors of an outbreak can have economic consequences and that response to an epidemic of foot-and-mouth disease "would involve the coordinated efforts of thousands of local, state and federal officials, and likely require the deployment of National Guard troops—and perhaps even federal troops to aid in the enforcement of quarantines and help destroy infected animals."

A *New York Times* report described a plot to smuggle the poison ricin into the food supply on at least one British military base in 2003.[4] The CIA had been following intelligence reports that a group of militants had devised a plan to use the poison on at least one military base in the United Kingdom. The United States wanted to know if one of Al Qaeda's leading experts on chemical and biological warfare was involved. Ricin was discovered in a London apartment during a raid in which four suspects were arrested. At least one of the suspects was believed to have been in contact with people who worked on at least one British military base. Ricin is taken from the castor bean and can be easily dissolved in a liquid or contained in a mist or powder. Consumed in any form, ricin causes stomach bleeding before attacking the spleen, liver, and kidneys and often causing death.

In early September 2003, the FBI issued a bulletin warning that terrorists might use two naturally occurring toxins, nicotine and solanine, to poison U.S. food or water supplies.[5] The FBI noted that terrorist manuals and documents recovered in Afghanistan refer to the use of these substances as poisons. Citing the supermarket employee who deliberately contaminated ground beef with an insecticide containing nicotine, FBI officials advised: "Such lone offenders, whether al-Qaida [sic] sympathizers or domestic criminals, are a concern to the FBI because they are so difficult to detect."

In 2003 during the World Cup race in New Zealand officials received letters purportedly from the "September 11" group threatening to use cyanide in food at the event. The letters referred to 25 kilograms of the poison purportedly stockpiled. The headlines read, "Cyanide Threat to Food, Warning: Watch What You Eat." Officials worried about cyanide spreading through the food supply and the number of deaths it could cause.

Caroline Smith DeWaal, JD, former director of food safety for the Center for Science in the Public Interest (CSPI), in 2004 wrote in *Food and Drug Law Journal* an analysis of policies affecting FDA-regulated products.[6] She feared that if a terrorist were to strike the U.S. food supply, consumer confidence in the government's fractured food safety programs would plummet as fast as confidence in airport security did following September 11.

DeWaal's report quoted Dr. John Bailar, chairman of the 1998 National Academy of Sciences (NAS) committee, writing three years later saying that "the 1998 NAS committee developed its recommendation based on the hazards that are already with us, paying almost no attention to bioterrorism. When bioterrorism is added to the mix, the case for prompt and sweeping change becomes compelling. While additional tinkering with the details of our food safety system might be helpful, the consolidation of responsibilities, authorities, and resources for food safety into a single high-level agency is critical."[7]

DeWaal warned, "Unfortunately, we live in a new era—one where we as Americans seem to be looking over our shoulders at all times. It is critical that the government is fully empowered to protect the public from potential biological, chemical and nuclear attack."

There's a relatively small department in the sprawling U.S. FDA bureaucracy with the ominous name of Office of Counterterrorism and Emerging Threats (OCET). One of its duties is preparation for and response to an attack involving biological agents, a complicated assignment due to the large number of potential agents, most of which are rarely encountered naturally. OCET must deal with potentially long incubation periods and consequent delayed onset of disease and the potential for secondary transmission. In addition to naturally occurring pathogens, agents used by bioterrorists may be genetically engineered to resist current therapies and evade vaccine-induced immunity. Pathogens that have been identified as potential biological warfare agents include those that cause anthrax, botulism, plague, smallpox, tularemia, and the hemorrhagic fevers, among others.

Threats to our food supply spread from farmlands and cattle ranches to our dinner table. Today, three agencies are involved in protecting our foods, both imported and domestically raised. Regulating and enforcing hundreds of rules and laws and reporting and investigating foodborne illnesses falls mainly to the USDA and the FDA. Repeated pleas and suggestions from lawmakers to consumer groups for one centralized food safety arm of government have been heard for years. But the status quo continues.

The U.S. Bioterrorism Act places more authority on U.S. Customs agents who are trained to conduct cargo and other examinations backed by laws that allow officers to hold suspect shipments for further examination and sampling. A prior notice must be submitted for any food imported or submitted for importation. The intent is to provide advance information to target potentially high-risk shipments that could threaten public health and the security of the food chain by an act of bioterrorism. Prior notice of imported foods must be received and confirmed electronically by the FDA no more than ten days before arrival in the United States and no fewer than two hours before arrival by land via road, four hours before arrival by air or by land via rail, or eight hours before arrival by water. The plan appears well thought out, but in reality there simply are not enough inspectors to get the job done.

In 2003, a study by RAND National Defense Research Group concluded that relatively little consideration has been paid to threats to the agriculture and food industries compared with transportation and telecommunications. RAND researcher Peter Chalk wrote about agroterrorism, which he described as "the deliberate introduction of a disease agent into the food chain, to undermine socioeconomic stability and/or generate fear."[8]

Painting a dire but important picture to consider, Chalk added, "A major agroterrorist attack would have substantial economic repercussions, especially when allied industries and services—suppliers, transporters, distributors, and restaurant chains—are taken into account. The fiscal downstream effect of a deliberate act of sabotage would be multidimensional, reverberating through other sectors of the economy and ultimately impacting the consumer."[9]

Aside from economic considerations, a successful bio-assault against the agricultural sector could also undermine the public's confidence in, and support for, the government. The mechanics of dealing with an attack—especially the potential need for mass animal slaughter to contain a major disease outbreak—could certainly generate public criticism (as it did during the 2001 foot-and-mouth epidemic in the United Kingdom).

Beyond the immediate economic and political impact, such attacks could also elicit fear and anxiety among the public. This would be particularly true in the event of a public health scare resulting from foodborne outbreaks or the spread of animal pathogens contagious to humans.

Former FBI director Robert Mueller as far back as 2005 said that terrorists have learned how to attack our food supply in some way. "We know that members of Al Qaeda have studied our agriculture industry."[10]

It didn't take the 9/11 attacks for the United States to prepare for biological and chemical attacks. The October 7, 2003, Risk Assessment for Food Terrorism report prepared by the Center for Food Safety and Applied Nutrition (CFSAN), an arm of the FDA, refers to terrorist attacks. The report outlines detailed preparations that were made in the 1990s, most of which are still in our strategic defense plans today. Some of the details are withheld because they contain classified information.

The U.S. Centers for Disease Control and Prevention (CDC) identified and ranked two foodborne pathogens as critical agents: Bacillus anthracis (anthrax) and Clostridium botulinum (botulism)—both of which are deadly pathogens and may contaminate food. Shigella dysenteriae, E. coli O157:H7, and ricin make up the next level of weapons in the form of deadly pathogens.[11] The CDC went a step further after identifying the most significant pathogens; it named certain chemicals that might be used in a terrorist attack on our food system. Those included heavy metals, such as arsenic, lead, and mercury, and the pesticides, dioxins, furans, and polychlorinated biphenyls (PCBs), all of which may be used to contaminate food. These toxins also have been introduced inadvertently into foods and linked to human health effects.

The CDC, in its strategic Plan for Preparedness and Response, issued this foreboding advisory: "Public health agencies must prepare also for the special features a terrorist attack probably would have."[12] "Terrorists might use combinations of these agents (methods), attack in more than one location simultaneously, use new agents, or use organisms that are not on the critical list (e.g., common, drug-resistant, or genetically engineered pathogens)."

As if that may not have been clear enough, the CDC wrote in the report:

> If an unintentional contamination of one food, such as clams, can affect 300,000 individuals, a concerted, deliberate attack on food could be devastating, especially if a more dangerous chemical, biological, or nuclear agent were used. It would be reasonable to assume that a terrorist using the food supply as a vehicle for attack would use an agent that would maximize the number of deaths associated with the contamination. Many of these agents are the same pathogens that have been linked to significant outbreaks of foodborne illness due to unintentional contamination. [13]

The World Health Organization contributed its warning: "The malicious contamination of food for terrorist purposes is a real and current threat." [14]

The CDC's infectious disease experts similarly have concluded that sabotage of food and water is the easiest means of biological or chemical attack largely because such attacks (albeit on a small scale) have been successful in the past. In addition, the CDC experts explain, the relative centralization of food production in the United States and the global distribution of food products give food a "unique susceptibility," and many points of vulnerability to sabotage intended to affect a large number of people exist in the food production and food distribution processes.

Another example of food sabotage can be drawn from a 1978 incident in which at least a dozen children in Holland and West Germany were hospitalized after a Middle East political group deliberately contaminated citrus fruit from Israel with mercury. Terrorists stated they were targeting the Israeli economy. [15]

Investigators say that the range of ways to conduct terroristic attacks on our food system is broad and their characteristics varied. They may include biological and chemical agents; naturally occurring, antibiotic-resistant, and genetically engineered substances; deadly agents and those tending to cause gastrointestinal discomfort; and highly infectious agents and those that are not communicable. Most sought-after substances readily include those available to any individual and those that are more difficult to acquire.

President Obama, addressing the UN General Assembly in 2011 said, "To lift the specter of mass destruction, we must come together to pursue the peace and security of a world without nuclear weapons. We must come together to prevent, detect, and fight every kind of biological danger, whether it is a pandemic like H1N1, a terrorist threat, or a treatable disease." [16]

One of the purposes of the 2011 FDA Food Safety Modernization Act (FSMA) is to better protect our food supply from intentional and unintentional contamination. Three years later, FSMA had not been funded by Congress and implemented by the White House. Described as landmark legislation, the law would give the FDA a modern mandate to improve the safety of our food. But instead, the United States is cutting back on enforcement, surveillance, and inspections of our imported food and in the food products we manufacture here.

Distinguishing a terrorist attack on our food poses a major concern, considering the many methods that could be used and from the many outbreaks of foodborne illnesses that occur every month in the United States. Determining intentional contamination of our food from unintentional causes of foodborne illnesses could take days, weeks, or even longer.

The eye-opening, shoot-from-the-hip CDC report on our susceptibility to a bioterrorism attack on our food supply concludes with this statement, issued more than a year before both the September 11 attacks and the anthrax incidents:

> An act of biological or chemical terrorism might range from dissemination of aerosolized anthrax spores to food product contamination, and predicting when and how such an attack might occur is not possible. However, the possibility of biological or chemical terrorism should not be ignored. . . . Preparing the nation to address this threat is a formidable challenge, but the consequences of being unprepared could be devastating.[17]

Where are we now? A CDC report in the summer of 2013 stated that the "United States is about a decade behind in building a national system for laboratories responding to chemical terrorism, compared to national bioterrorism activities."[18]

Chapter Two

Food Imports

Our increasing appetites for imported foods and spices grow every year, but our poor efforts to insure that the foods we bring into this country are safe continue to fail miserably. Here are some mind-boggling facts: The United States imports more than 80 percent of seafood consumed in this country, about 40 percent of fruit and nuts, and 20 percent of our fresh vegetables. More than 10 million food shipments arrive at 300 different U.S. ports from over 300,000 factories in 150 different countries each year. The average American eats about 260 pounds of imported foods annually. That's about 13 percent of our diet.[1]

In 2008 the National Institutes of Health (NIH) concluded, "Rightly or wrongly, imported food is held responsible for the greatest risks" to the foods we eat.[2] Importing infectious disease along with food can be a source of danger involving multiple agents, mainly bacteria but also parasites.

Despite that firm warning, the FDA describes its inspection of foods arriving from nearly 200 countries at 300 different ports of entry as simply "inadequate." Worried food safety watchdogs call the inspections virtually nonexistent. The FDA maintains a list of high-priority sites overseas but inspects only 11 percent of those facilities each year.

Some of the cases of disease outbreaks linked to imported foods have been compiled by the PEW Health Group:[3]

- Fifty-two Americans were hospitalized and nearly 300 more were sickened across 44 states after eating salami coated with black and red pepper contaminated with Salmonella montevideo.[4] The pepper was imported from three Asian countries in 2009 and 2010.

- Two people died, nearly 300 others were hospitalized, and almost 1,500 were sickened in 43 states after consuming Salmonella saintpaul-contaminated serrano and jalapeno peppers imported from Mexico in 2008.[5]
- Sixteen people were hospitalized and 51 sickened throughout 16 states after eating cantaloupe contaminated with Salmonella litchfield. Honduras shipped the melons into the United States in 2008.[6]
- In 2007, a Chinese ingredient supplier to pet food companies in North America used a dangerous substance in its product to save money, according to the FDA:[7] melamine, an animal feed filler that, when combined with another chemical, cyanuric acid, causes kidney failure.[8] After issuing a recall, which encompassed 100 brands of pet food, the FDA received 18,000 phone calls from consumers reporting their pet's illness.

The PEW Health Group makes strong recommendations to the FDA every year:[9]

- The FDA should build a robust inspection program relating to inspection of foreign facilities.
- The FDA must balance resources for both foreign and domestic inspections.
- The FDA should leverage inspection resources of other federal agencies.
- The FDA should rely more on inspections made by trusted foreign governments.
- The FDA should demonstrate that all importers must play by the rules or suffer consequences.
- Third-party audits must be required with complete transparency.

These are strong words that bring few results each year. Food safety experts see little, if any, change in the FDA's role of inspecting imported food. The United States inspected less than 2 percent of food imported from China, while conducting only 13 inspections of China's many food production facilities over a 12-month period in 2009–2010.[10] The problem deepens when we learn that more than half the Chinese food processing and packaging firms failed that country's own safety inspections in 2011. China continues experiencing critical food outbreaks and scandals.

Honey, contaminated in China with heavy metals and animal antibiotics, finds its way to grocery shelves throughout the United States. Millions of pounds of Chinese honey reach our stores after first being transshipped to India and Vietnam, according to *Ethical Foods*.[11] The European Union (EU), made up of 28 countries, banned the illegal honey shipped from India. But the tainted Chinese honey continues to pour into the United States with no action from our government to stop the imports.

Import Genius, a shipping intelligence service commissioned by Food Safety News, provides interesting facts from its databases of all U.S. Customs import sites:

- The United States imported 208 million pounds of honey over the past 18 months.
- About 48 million pounds came from trusted and usually reliable suppliers in Argentina, Brazil, Canada, Uruguay, and Mexico.
- Almost 60 percent of what was imported—123 million pounds—came from Asian countries, traditional laundering points for Chinese honey. This included 45 million pounds from India alone. [12]
- China's food safety problems are massive and include the sale of diseased ducks to unsuspecting customers, pork deliberately laced with chemicals, and tainted milk that killed six babies and sickened 300,000 other people. China's National People's Congress reported in 2011 that almost 300 people who violated serious food safety laws received penalties of life in prison or the death penalty. [13]

The Chinese people wait in fear for the next food scandal and wonder where it might hit. Grace Ng, a writer for the Asia News Network, reported that no deaths or mass poisoning cases have been directly linked to the latest bout of food scandals. [14] "But they have nonetheless heightened public jitters," she adds. "It's not that nothing is being done, but enforcement improvements represent only a beginning."

Chinese officials in Beijing and Shanghai promise a crackdown starting with a plan to blacklist manufacturing and packaging companies violating food safety laws. The planned laws, which were to be released in 2014, will block companies caught using banned substances in food or illegally producing and selling banned food additives from operating in the two cities, according to the news agency Xinhua.

Food safety inspectors in China confirm 15,000 cases of food safety violations in a six-month period in 2012. During that time, the government closed 5,700 unlicensed food service establishments. One of the major complaints in China being heard from a more vocal citizenry is the use of cooking oil that's made by reprocessing used oil. The product has been referred to as "gutter oil." In early 2012, China's Ministry of Public Security reported 100 arrests in a massive crackdown on gang-related illegal cooking oil producers. [15] The suspects used rotten animal carcasses and internal organs along with waste fat to produce the cooking oil. The number of arrests by early 2013 leveled off at 350. China's State Food and Drug Administration wants stronger laws regulating the use of non-food substances, including poppy capsules and powder, antibiotics to season beverages and flavorings, and

Sudan red, an azo dye. Sudan red is used in turpentine-based polishes and some hair dyes.

A scathing report, produced in 2013 by the Research Laboratory and Crisis Management Center of Shanghai Jiao Tong University, pointed to private companies most often linked to food safety scandals in 2012 at 53 percent of the total, compared with 17 percent by multinational companies. [16] Here are some of the findings:

- In February 2012, frozen dumpling producer Zhengzhou Sinian Food Co. in Henan province suffered a loss of public confidence after a customer found an adhesive bandage inside a glutinous rice dumpling. [17]
- In April, preserved fruits sold by several big-brand stores, including snack chains Laiyifen and Baiweilin, were processed in unsanitary factories and had excessive additives. [18] All are private companies.
- In December, the Shanghai Food Safety Office said excessive amounts of antibiotics were found in eight batches of raw chicken samples taken from a KFC supplier from 2010 to 2011, triggering public outrage. [19]

China's food industry suffered a crisis of confidence in 2008, when milk powder produced by a company in Hebei province was illegally laced with melamine. [20] The chemical additive led to the deaths of six children and sickened 300,000 others, according to the report.

By 2013, the USDA began pointing to increased attention the FDA is giving to food imports from China as an indicator of its concern about food safety with those products. China's weak enforcement of food safety laws and its policy of allowing heavy use of agricultural chemicals increase the safety risks. Since the FDA inspects only a small number of shipments from China, it's not surprising that it has found food items contaminated with unsafe additives, improper food processing and handling in fish and shellfish, and what the agency describes quite appropriately as just plain "filth." [21]

Despite India's implication in Chinese honey smuggling, I found one positive approach to the food safety problem. Tough new laws enacted by the Food Safety and Standards Authority of India require that sick and unfit food handlers must pass mandatory medical tests and demonstrate their fitness for work. Additionally, the workers must pass an eye test and skin examination and be vaccinated against an enteric group of diseases.

Ghanaian health officials appear to be moving out of the dark ages in dealing with food safety. Nurevas, a new food-processing company in Accra, will adhere to the highest European standards by using state-of-the-art equipment and the ability to trace the origin of all foods.

In 2011, Interpol-Europol seized hundreds of tons of fake and dangerously substandard foods including cheese, tea, and olive oil, breaking up a major organized criminal operation stretching across ten countries. [22] Tons of expired meat discovered in a Beirut warehouse led to the arrest of 20 people and the filing of criminal charges of premeditated attempted murder.

The FDA maintains full-time inspectors at only 90 of the 300 U.S. ports of entry. Importers know inspectors at these ports are few and far between and check only 1 percent of the food shipments. If importers should fail an inspection at one port, they know they can go to the next port where the odds are heavily weighed on their side to move freely through the port of entry without an inspection.

The CDC warns that foodborne disease outbreaks caused by imported food rise every year. Significantly, nearly half of the outbreaks traced to imported foods are from areas that previously had not been associated with outbreaks. The result of our lax and substandard inspections, enforcements, and seizures allow potentially deadly pathogens in contaminated foods to reach our dinner tables unabated.[23]

Fish and spices top the list of foods most likely to cause problems. Since the late 1990s the amount of imported food reaching the United States doubled, according to the CDC. The number of outbreaks mirrors that increase.

Hannah Gould, an epidemiologist in CDC's Division of Foodborne, Waterborne, and Environmental Diseases, put it this way: "As our food supply becomes more global, people are eating foods from all over the world, potentially exposing them to germs from all corners of the world, too."[24] "We saw an increased number of outbreaks due to imported foods during recent years, and more types of foods from more countries causing outbreaks."[25]

Thanks are due to our many professional investigative reporters for their continuing efforts in digging out hidden facts directly affecting food safety in the United States. Helena Bottemiller with Food Safety News (www.foodsafetynews.com) discovered that the USDA in late 2012 quietly eliminated 60 percent of foreign meat inspections.[26] That means the USDA drastically sliced a major investigative component that has long been established to inspect meat and poultry at its source, prior to shipment to the United States.[27] Ms. Bottemiller found that "the USDA's Food Safety and Inspection Service has also become less transparent. The agency failed to make audit reports public in a timely fashion and revealed which countries have been audited in the past two years only after multiple inquiries by Food Safety News."[28]

The U.S. government urgently needs a law to prosecute importers of bad food, but instead, real criminal penalties have been cut from proposed new laws, according to Jaydee Hanson, a senior policy analyst at the Center for Food Safety.[29]

Why does the FDA allow orange juice containing the fungicide carbendazim to be imported from Brazil, when in 2009 the United States banned the chemical for use in this country? It's another case of the FDA siding with industry over safety issues. "We think it would be unduly disruptive of the food supply to try to withdraw that product from the market," says FDA deputy director Michael Taylor. Instead of a strictly enforced ban, the FDA simply imposed a limit on the amount of carbendazim that can be contained in orange juice imported from Brazil.[30] Carbendazim on citrus in the United States had been illegal but commonly used in Brazil to combat mold on orange trees. It is permitted up to a limit in imports to the European Union, the main buyer of Brazil's juice.

We live in a global community when it comes to imports and exports. One of the best examples comes from Patrick Wall, associate professor of Public Health in University College Dublin's School of Public and Population Sciences: "We catch fish in Scotland, fly it five thousand miles to China where it's shelled by hand, then we fly it five thousand miles back to Scotland where it's sold as 'fresh'." In an interview with Australian Food News, Wall said, "Regulation means nothing if it's not enforced properly. Australia applies more controls over the food chain than the European Union (EU)."[31] More than two dozen countries now belong to the EU.

European nations are far ahead of the United States because those countries making up the EU strictly enforce their own import standards and regulations. Here's a terrific example from *Food Quality and Safety*: "Companies based in the U.S. and other non-European nations must comply [to our laws] if they wish to continue selling in Europe. This means that for a candy bar to be shelved in a Paris grocery store, its Illinois-based candy manufacturer must be able to identify which North Carolina farm grew the peanuts inside the bar."[32]

One more thing before we move on to fruits, vegetables, and the diseases they attract. In all of this unprecedented development of the food industry and food trade in the world, rightly or wrongly, imported food is held responsible for the greatest risks. As said earlier, importing an infectious disease along with food can be a source of danger, involving multiple agents, mainly bacterial (Salmonella, campylobacter, verotoxin-producing Escherichia coli, Listeria), but also parasitic (Toxoplasma gondii, Cyclospora cayetanensis, Trichinella spp), and viral (norovirus, Hepatitis A virus), as well as nonconventional communicable agents and mycotoxins. Prevention of food risks means enforcing international regulations on the part of the 149 member states of the World Trade Organization (WTO) and increasing vigilance with regard to illegal imports of food, systematically investigating collective foodborne outbreaks, and finally implementing controls according to the hazard analysis and critical control point (HACCP) method.

The food safety problems associated with imported foods are not new issues. But they are issues growing exponentially over the years, creating potentially fatal consequences of fast-expanding proportions. During my research, a headline in the *New York Times* caught my eye: "Tainted Imports—

Special Report: Imports Swamp Food-Safety Efforts." The story was published on September 29, 1997. Look at the opening line of the article:

> Since the 1980s, food imports to the United States have doubled. But Federal inspections of those imports by the FDA have dropped to less than half what they were five years ago."[33]

That article correctly cited a major food safety issue from years ago, and it not only holds true decades later, the problem worsened.

Chapter Three

Produce

THE VITAL PATHOGEN-TESTING PROGRAM
THAT IS NO LONGER

It's not a common household subject, not even ranking as one of the top ten well-known food safety programs. But the Microbiological Data Program (MDP) could be considered the benchmark for taxpayers to demand government always provide the most bang for the buck.[1] Operating on a relatively small budget, $4.5 million from a $3 trillion budget, it collected and analyzed data on foodborne pathogens on high-risk fruits and vegetables.[2] Samples were taken at markets and chain store distribution centers in various parts of the nation. Labs performed analytical testing for specific pathogens. Results could trigger nationwide recalls.

But now it's dead, buried, forgotten. The only such program in the United States that worked, playing a major role keeping most of the food pathogens in fruits and vegetables from reaching our dinner tables, is now in our rearview mirrors. The fierce lobbyists for the United Fresh Produce Association, the Big Daddy of the corporate fruit and vegetable growers, sliced the life out of the program in 2012.[3] The politics behind the move couldn't be hidden. The program, initiated in the George Bush presidency, has been ended by the Obama administration.[4]

The *Huffington Post* said the budget cut removed a key entity that "can trigger nationwide recalls, and keep tainted produce from reaching consumers or grocery store shelves." The article also pointed out that industry leaders from the United Fresh Produce Association repeatedly pushed the government to get rid of the testing program, saying it had cost growers millions of dollars in produce recalls.[5]

As of early 2012, the federal program had tested high-risk produce such as alfalfa sprouts, cilantro, green onions, peppers, tomatoes, spinach, and other leafy greens. "Every one of these vegetables has caused a foodborne illness outbreak or recall over the years, some of them lethal thanks in part to an industrialized food system that transports bugs nationwide," according to Michele Simon, a public health lawyer specializing in food industry marketing and lobbying tactics.[6] She's the author of *Appetite for Profit: How the Food Industry Undermines Our Health and How to Fight Back* and *A Budget Cut Only the Produce Industry Could Love*.

In July 2011, the *Chicago Tribune* touted the positive effects of the MDP. "Over the last two years, MDP findings have triggered at least 19 produce recalls," according to the FDA. During its 11-year run, the MDP conducted 80 percent of all federal produce testing for pathogens like *Salmonella* and *Listeria*.[7] The program, created under President George W. Bush and his 2001 Food Safety Initiative, tested thousands of samples of fruits and vegetables each year, gathered from 11 distribution centers.[8]

We have lost sight of food safety when it comes to the fruits and vegetables we eat. Most of the outbreaks and recalls are directed at contaminated produce, both imported from Mexico and other countries and those grown here in the United States. Here, fresh produce accounts for almost half of all foodborne illnesses each year. The USDA must provide more help, not less. The proof lies in the summer of 2013, when the parasite Cyclospora sickened more than 500 people in 16 states.

Most people infected with Salmonella develop diarrhea, fever, and abdominal cramps 12 to 72 hours after infection. Illnesses usually last four to seven days, and many people recover without treatment, according to the FDA.

However, in some victims, the diarrhea may be so severe that the patient needs to be hospitalized. In these patients, the Salmonella infection may spread from the intestines to the blood stream, and then to other body sites and can cause death unless the person is treated promptly with antibiotics.[9] Salmonellosis strikes children more than adults. The rate of diagnosed infections in children younger than five years old is higher than the rate in all other persons. Young children, the elderly, and those with compromised immune systems are the most likely to have severe infections. More than 400 persons die each year in the United States as a result of acute Salmonellosis.[10]

DISEASES AND OUTBREAKS

One of the largest Salmonellosis outbreaks in the United States since 1985 hit in the spring of 2008, spreading across 44 states and sickening 1,442 people. The Salmonella saintpaul-tainted jalapeno and serrano peppers from Mexico caused at least one death and hospitalized 257 others, according to the CDC.

The outbreak strain was isolated from samples of jalapeno peppers collected in a U.S. warehouse, at a patient's home, and from samples of serrano peppers and water collected on a farm in Mexico.[11]

Cantaloupes, proven to be susceptible to various pathogens, were the vehicles for Listeria, Hepatitis A, and Salmonella illnesses. Jensen Farms cantaloupes killed 23 people and sickened 147 others in 28 states in 2011 in one of the deadliest outbreaks of foodborne illness in U.S. history.[12]

The FDA says Listeria monocytogenes contaminated cantaloupe grown in the production fields near Granada, Colorado.[13] In August 2012 the FDA recalled cantaloupes grown by Chamberlain Farms of Owensville, Indiana, due to possible contamination with Salmonella typhimurium.[14] The sickness spread across 21 states, infecting 178 people.

Salmonella panama–contaminated fresh cantaloupe from Del Monte Fresh Produce N.A., Inc., sickened 13 people in five states in 2011.[15]

It was the Salmonella litchfield strain that made 51 people sick across 16 states in April 2008.[16] Cantaloupe imported from Agropecuaria Montelibano, a Honduran company, was cited as the likely source of the illnesses, according to the CDC.[17]

Additionally, in 2011, 60 people in ten states became ill from an E. coli O157:H7 outbreak linked to romaine lettuce.[18] At least 30 people were hospitalized and two developed severe kidney disease. The CDC did not name the supplier but referred to "Farm A."[19]

Many of these cases show how the U.S. government leaves the impression that it is protecting big business before they protect the consumer with its foot-dragging and secrecy regarding public information about enforcement, closures, and seizures.

PricewaterhouseCoopers put it perfectly with this warning: "Optimizing produce food safety is simply good business."[20]

Many of our exported fruits and vegetables have been banned in some countries because of our poor food safety standards. Foremost are spinach and peanut butter. When you're sickened from eating either of these foods, Salmonella usually is the culprit. If other countries with a more progressive food safety inspection program say "no" to some of our foods, who are we to say "yes" to government inspection agencies like the FDA and USDA, with dubious intentions in food safety enforcement policies that appear to continually favor the food producer and manufacturer?

In 2008, Keebler and Austin brands of peanut butter crackers were contaminated with Salmonella typhimurium, which sickened 714 in 46 states.[21]

Trader Joe's Valencia peanut butter, manufactured by Sunland, Inc., led to an outbreak that infected 42 persons with the strain of Salmonella bredeney in 20 states.[22] On November 26, 2012, the FDA suspended Sunland's registration and prohibited the company from providing food products for sale to the public.[23]

Salmonella causes diarrhea and fever resulting in Salmonellosis, which kills more than 400 people a year in the United States.

Taylor Farms, linked to part of the Cyclospora parasite outbreak in 2013, fielded other problems that same year.[24] The company instituted a nationwide, voluntary recall of organic baby spinach products over concerns it may have been contaminated with E.coli, according to the FDA.[25]

Alfalfa sprouts carried Salmonella two years in a row. In 2009 the consumption of sprouts contaminated with Salmonella saintpaul sickened 235 people in 14 states.[26] The patients ranged in age from one to 85 years. Seeds sold by the Caudill Seed Company of Louisville, Kentucky, are believed to have been the source of the contamination. A spokesman for the company, Lyle Orwig, quoted in news reports, said at the time of the outbreak that the seeds were imported from Italy and sold at various facilities throughout the United States.[27]

A year later, and about the time of a romaine lettuce outbreak, 140 people in 27 states came down with Salmonellosis after consuming alfalfa sprouts sold at Wal-Mart stores, Trader Joe's, and Caldwell Fresh Foods.[28] The chances of Salmonella contaminating sprouts increase because they're grown in a warm, humid environment. Food safety experts stated at the time that there had been more than two dozen outbreaks of foodborne illnesses linked to sprouts, according to the *Huffington Post*.[29]

Cantaloupes are not the only fruit to be hit hard by pathogens that cause foodborne illnesses. Imported Salmonella agona–contaminated papayas sickened 106 people in 25 states in 2011, sending at least 10 of the victims to hospitals.[30] Agromod Produce, Inc., located a few miles north of the Texas-Mexico border near McAllen, Texas, distributed the papayas, imported from Mexico.

The sickness spread to 25 states due to the nationwide distribution of the papayas to wholesalers and retailers and to Canada. People sickened ranged in age from younger than one to 91, and the median age was 20.[31]

Another nationwide recall of imported fruit from Mexico involved the Daniella brand of mangoes contaminated with Salmonella braenderup.[32] The fruit sickened 105 people in 16 states.[33] The California Department of Public Health reported 73 cases, the largest number in the United States. Typically, mangoes have a shelf life of five to eight days after they're sold. About 900,000 mangoes containing high levels of arsenic were shipped across the country under several brand names to hundreds of grocery stores including most major supermarket chains, slowing the recall process.[34]

USA Today's investigation concluded that the fruit was grown by Agricola Daniela, a large grower near the town of Ahome, on the coast of the Sea of Cortez in the northwestern part of the Mexican state of Sinaloa.[35]

Amid scores of complaints from consumers and food safety advocates, the FDA, after two years of pressure, lowered the allowed levels of inorganic arsenic from 23 parts per billion (ppb) to 10 ppb, which is the same level set by the U.S. Environmental Protection Agency (EPA) for arsenic in drinking water.[36] Inorganic arsenic has been linked to cardiovascular disease and diabetes.[37] *Consumer Reports* recommended a 3 ppb limit.[38]

You might ask, and rightfully so, "If our government isn't fully protecting us, what do we do?" Our government agencies—FDA, USDA, and CDC— have some free advice:

- Thoroughly wash fruits and vegetables. Scrub, not just wash, the hard skin products such as avocados, watermelons, and cantaloupes. Yes, you're going to peel them and, yes, your knife first comes in contact with the outer skin and picks up any contaminate on its way to the meat of the produce. So, wash and scrub.
- Wash and scrub your hands. The correct way is washing 15 seconds with soap and water and rinsing another 15 seconds. Why rinse for 15 seconds? Soap has germs, too.
- Know the fruits and veggies with the most pesticides, and take extra caution and care dealing with these products. In fact, treat all of them as such.

Almost half of all foodborne illnesses that led to hospitalization or death between 1998 and 2008 were attributable to fresh produce, according to the CDC.[39] "While fresh fruits and vegetables are the cornerstone to a healthy diet, improperly handled they can be literally lethal," a March 2013 CDC report states.[40]

In 1984 Earthbound Farms began operations with a 2½-acre raspberry farm in California's Carmel Valley. Drew and Myra Goodman, determined young transplants from the towering skyscrapers of Manhattan, eagerly scooped up their first shovels of soil.[41] They did just about everything right, building those 2½ acres into the country's largest grower of organic produce.

Will Daniels, senior vice president of operations at Earthbound, had some interesting observations at the 2013 annual meeting of the Food Safety Summit Expo in Baltimore.[42] "Grocery retailers routinely put profits above food safety, preferring to save money via bypassing initiatives that could keep shoppers safer in order to pad their bottom line," Daniels said.[43]

"We must stop thinking that it's OK to roll the risk-aversion dice in an effort to save money," Daniels said. "If food safety is not a competitive advantage, then every company should be happy to share their success."

Several years later, after it was linked to an E. coli outbreak from its spinach, Earthbound Farm implemented a "multiple-hurdle" system that sends the product through rigorous "test-and-hold" procedures in the raw and finished stages.[44]

But few in the industry copied the Earthbound model, claiming it is expensive and unreliable. That bothers Daniels, who says other companies have not followed Earthbound simply because they're more concerned about profit than safety. "We believed—and still believe to this day—that what we are doing is the right thing for fresh-cut produce and the risk associated with our products and our distribution. Why aren't more people following us?"[45]

Meanwhile, inspectors often are seen as enemy agents only looking to penalize or close companies, rather than help the industry upgrade its food safety efforts. Retailers and grower-shippers go on the defensive when inspectors show up, Daniels said. What should be happening is a collaborative effort between produce purveyors and inspectors to shore up the industry's food safety efforts. A few days after Daniels's speech, Reuters news agency reported that Earthbound Farm had made contact with an officer at Barclays Bank to find a buyer.[46]

Chapter Four

Poultry

Something is sadly and dangerously wrong when the government turns its back when chicken laced with Salmonella is found during processing at a Foster Farms plant in California.[1] "Cockroaches were also found at this Foster Farms plant by federal inspectors on September 14, 2013,[2] November 4, 2013, December 28, 2013, and January 7, 2014,"[3] according to the USDA.[4] Cockroaches were "observed and documented on multiple days (including on two consecutive days) in multiple locations within the establishment." The USDA contaminated chickens continue to roll off the production lines and be packaged, shipped, and placed in stores for us to buy, cook, eat, and make us sick.

In 2013, more than 400 people were poisoned from eating the Salmonella-adulterated chicken. Inspectors visited the Foster Farms plant a few months later, discovered a few cockroaches at the same plant, and immediately ordered a halt to all production.

So many of our federal food safety laws and rules are written to favor the industry far above the safety of the public. Inspectors are restricted from ordering a shutdown of a plant and requiring a recall when Salmonella-contaminated chicken is discovered because Salmonella is "naturally occurring and not an adulterant." The laws allow the FDA to drag its feet on issues that would protect consumers but adversely affect big business, like ignoring the public for four years before banning most arsenic-based drugs fed to turkeys and chickens. Budgets, kept far below needed levels, prevent most of the testing and surveillance that's required. Some food production facilities receive a visit from an inspector once every 10 years or more due to the shortage of inspectors.

Salmonella affects at least 42,000 people across the United States every year.[5] The CDC says most of the Salmonella-related illnesses go unreported and the actual number of people sickened could be 30 times higher or more than a million people stricken.[6] Symptoms include fever, cramps, and diarrhea.

A *Consumer Reports* study in 2013 found 97 percent of raw chicken breasts tested were laced with bacteria that could make you sick or worse.[7] Chicken was purchased at various stores across the country, and 316 chicken breasts were tested, including some labeled organic. "Harmful bacteria was lurking in almost all the chicken," according to the report. "More deaths are attributed to poultry than to any other commodity," according to the CDC.

We are told repeatedly by government agencies that cooking chicken to 165 degrees Fahrenheit kills all Salmonella.[8] In October 2013 the news media across the country carried stories about how Costco cooked its rotisserie chicken to at least 180 degrees Fahrenheit, but Salmonella heidelberg, a strain of the pathogen illnesses, remained in some of the birds.[9]

USE OF ANTIBIOTICS WITH ANIMALS

Here's another problem: Public health officials state unequivocally that resistance to antibiotics has reached a critical level. Because many meat-producing farms use subclinical antibiotics in an effort to keep animals "healthy," the animals, and the bacteria they contract, have built up resistance to these antibiotics, becoming superbugs of a sort. These bugs can then infect humans who work with the animals or others who come in contact. The CDC calls the problem a dire threat to our health, citing the fact that antibiotic-resistant infections are linked to at least two million illnesses and 23,000 deaths in the United States each year. Simply stated, using antibiotics creates resistance.[10] Animals that receive antibiotics develop resistant bacteria in their guts. Drug-resistant bacteria can remain on meat from animals. When not handled or cooked properly, the bacteria can spread to humans. Also, fertilizers and water containing animal feces and drug-resistant bacteria are used on food crops. Drug-resistant bacteria in the animal feces can remain on crops and be eaten. These bacteria can remain in the human gut, according to the CDC.[11]

In February 2014, the city of Providence, Rhode Island, made history when it became the first U.S. city to take action against the misuse of antibiotics on factory farms.[12] Led by Councilman Seth Yurdin, the City Council passed a resolution asking federal lawmakers to restrict antibiotics for human use only. Calling the issue a public health crisis, the councilmen called for an immediate halt in the use of antibiotics in animal feed. The measure calls for every member of Rhode Island's congressional delegation to support any legislation that would ban the misuse of all antibiotics on factory farms. But, it's only a resolution. No teeth.

The temporary solution for consumers is simply to select chicken raised without the use of antibiotics and purchase poultry from farmers who keep their chickens off unnecessary drugs, preserving the effectiveness of antibiotics, according to *Consumer Reports*. Of course, don't forget all those safe food-handling requirements that we'll cover in detail in another chapter.

ARSENIC AND OLD LACE CHICKEN

The FDA released some interesting yet tepid news in 2013. The agency banned the use of most arsenic-laced drugs that have been fed to turkeys and chickens for years by many producers to promote growth and prevent disease.[13] The ban on all but three arsenic-based drugs did not come without foot dragging by the government and many legal and public pressures. For four years the FDA ignored pleas from the public and from food safety watchdog groups calling for bans on all animal drugs containing arsenic.

The FDA refused to revoke the license for nitarsone, which also contains arsenic, until "more research is completed."[14] Will that take another four years?

While the kind of arsenic fed to animals cannot be categorized as a carcinogen, after the contaminated feed is eaten by the chickens and turkeys it is converted to a form that suggests it is a cancer-causing agent. This may be one of the main reasons the FDA, after a few years, banned most of the arsenic-bearing animal drugs.

Bloomberg News published an interesting progression, saying, "Just as troubling as evidence that trace arsenic might be in the meat we eat is what happens to the toxin once it is passed through as animal waste. Some of the waste is used as fertilizer, or isn't properly disposed of, leading to arsenic in soil, water, and crops."[15]

"The real mystery here is why the FDA just can't bring itself to do what it deemed necessary more than a generation ago," author James Grieff wrote in *Bloomberg*.[16] So, next time you hear someone worrying that the 2013 government shutdown had caused the agency to stop functioning, you can reassure them with the fact that, even when fully funded, the FDA isn't keeping us all that safe.

When attempting to understand the very real concerns about arsenic in chicken, we need to look at the history of the U.S. government's first approval of the use of arsenic in chicken feed.[17] Producers started using arsenicals back in the 1940s when they discovered they could make more money by promoting faster growth and treating disease at the same time. No one raised a question about the safety of the practice, which became standard in the industry by 2010.[18] It was estimated that 88 percent of all chickens raised for food in the United States were given roxarsone, an arsenic-based drug, now banned.

Scientists at the Johns Hopkins Center for a Livable Future exposed the facts about chickens being fed arsenic in their food in a paper published in May 2013.[19] Researchers collected samples from grocery stores in 10 cities across the country. Some USDA-certified organic and "antibiotic-free" products were included. The scientists found chicken meat samples contained up to three times more arsenic than a maximum level proposed by the FDA in 2011. The FDA later withdrew that proposal.

Chris Hunt wrote about the study in May 2013: "The study showed that chickens likely raised with arsenic-based drugs yield meat that has higher levels of inorganic arsenic, a known carcinogen that has also been associated with cardiovascular disease, type 2 diabetes, cognitive deficits, and adverse pregnancy."[20]

The United States produces 8.7 billion broiler chickens each year, with at least 70 percent having been fed arsenic.[21] Arsenic doesn't degrade or disappear, but it helps contaminate much of the 45 billion pounds of litter and waste generated each year by the American chicken industry. A study by the Institute for Agriculture and Trade Policy examined the house dust in 31 homes in the chicken-producing town of Prairie Grove, Arkansas.[22] Every one of the 31 homes tested was found to contain at least two kinds of arsenic also found in chicken litter.

The study also points out that arsenic levels in chicken meat are much higher than previously acknowledged. That was the conclusion of USDA scientists writing in 2004 in *Environmental Health Perspectives*, a journal of the National Institutes of Health.

An interesting fact in this study anticipated an argument that if you cook the chicken well, the arsenic will disappear. Wrong. Researchers cut each sample in half and cooked one half, leaving the other half raw. The cooked samples had higher levels of inorganic arsenic than the uncooked half.[23]

In 2008, Russia began banning U.S.-raised chickens due to excess of arsenic and the presence of E.coli and Salmonella.[24]

So why did the FDA wait so long, four years or more, to prohibit arsenicals from chickens produced for food? Perhaps the hesitation can be traced to our government's leaning toward protecting big business rather than protecting the health of Americans. What's being done on the many other fronts dealing with protecting our health when eating chicken and turkey?

Allowing the fox to guard the hen house may be one way to save money, but when it comes to poultry inspections, the results could be extremely serious and potentially deadly.

The USDA wants to expand a pilot program that puts most of the inspection responsibilities in the hands of the private processors, eliminating up to 800 inspector positions, which reduces the number of federal inspectors from four to only one on conveyor lines where the birds are checked.[25] And that lone agent would be at the end of the line. The conveyor line speed would increase, sending 170 birds a minute past that single inspector, rather than the current 130 birds a minute inspected by four agents.

The USDA claims checking for defective chickens should be the responsibility of the poultry producers and processors.[26] In early April 2012, nearly 100 inspectors opposed to the new proposal picketed the USDA facility in Washington carrying signs; one sign read "Chicken Inspection Isn't a Speed Sport."[27] The inspectors warn the new regulation would put the public at greater risk.

Food & Water Watch, a nonprofit, public interest organization, checked out what was going on inside a USDA experimental program known as the Hazard Analysis and Critical Control Points (HACCP) Inspection Models Project. As our bureaucratic system would have it, within HACCP the USDA created HIMP, which stands for the HACCP Inspection Models Project. HIMP tests the idea of allowing poultry processors to monitor their own operations. Food & Water Watch "found evidence of food contamination in many of the test slaughter facilities, including bits of beak, feathers, lungs, oil glands, bile, and even fecal matter still on carcasses after the employee inspection."[28] In 2011, some of the chicken facilities' average error rate was 64 percent, but increased to between 87 and 100 percent in turkey slaughter facilities.

In April 2012, ABC News produced a major investigative report titled "USDA to Let Industry Self-Inspect Chicken."[29] The network pointed out that it has an average audience of seven million viewers each night. In the report, Food Safety and Inspection Service (FSIS) inspector Stan Painter told ABC News that HIMP plants fudge test results by tweaking processes "when they know a test is coming" to make the program look better.

In a prepared statement, published in April 2012 by the *Huffington Post*, Al Almanza, administrator of the FSIS of the USDA, said: "Some in the debate have said that we are turning over inspection to the industry to determine what is safe for consumers. Nothing could be more misleading or incorrect. USDA inspectors will be in every plant, ensuring the safety of these products, and the proportion of them doing critical food safety related tasks will actually increase. In the 34 years of my career focused on food safety, I have seen—again and again—the need to modernize to keep up with the latest science and threats. This poultry slaughter modernization proposal is about protecting public health, plain and simple."[30] Food & Water Watch issued a statement saying, "Cutting the budget does not justify putting the health and safety of consumers and workers in the balance."

Before I talk about one of my favorite writers, Marion Nestle, I need to lay some groundwork. "Pink slime" is a term coined by USDA microbiologist Gerald Zirnstein in 2002 to describe the leftover fatty bits that are spun around at a high temperature in an ammonia solution to kill E. coli and other bacteria.[31] From there it's mixed into the ground beef that is ready for packaging and shipment. Now, we have "Toxic Chicken Is the New Pink Slime," the headline to an article in one of the most respected publications in America, *The Atlantic*. The story is a concise and thorough investigative story by Marion Nestle, who publishes food safety articles on her website, www.FoodPolitics.com.[32] Highly respected in food safety circles, Ms. Nestle has written numerous books about food industry politics and food safety and has a PhD in molecular biology.

She gathers some of the most vital information she can find and sets out to show what other writers and experts are saying about the USDA plan. As Dana Milbank of the *Washington Post* puts it, it's "a proposal to allow chicken slaughterhouses to inspect themselves—eliminating those pesky federal monitors who have the annoying habit of taking diseased birds out of the food supply. Even if the Obama administration were inclined to bring down capitalism with an orgy of overregulation, there isn't enough money in the budget to enforce the rules on the books. That's what the chicken fight is about: Spending cuts . . . are a form of de facto deregulation."[33]

The *New York Times* account of this policy change notes that inspectors "had observed numerous instances of poultry plant employees allowing birds contaminated with fecal matter or other substances to pass.[34] And even when the employees try to remove diseased birds, they face reprimands. The Agriculture Department proposal allows poultry plants to speed up their assembly lines to about 200 birds per minute from 140, hampering efforts to examine birds for defects."[35]

The Center for a Livable Future at Johns Hopkins reports that meal made from chicken by-products (in this case, feathers) contains arsenic and antibiotics such as fluoroquinolones that have been banned by the FDA for use in poultry, according to Ms. Nestle. A study published in *Environmental Science & Technology* found fluoroquinolone antibiotics in 8 of 12 samples of feather meal collected from six states and China. A second study found arsenic in every sample of feather meal tested. These findings indicate that poultry producers are using these drugs, even though they are not allowed to do so.

Ms. Nestle wraps up her article with this: "I don't know what the best system for inspection might be, but I'm quite sure that leaving food safety oversight to the discretion of the packers is not a good idea. Neither is speeding up the line. And neither is feeding chickens drugs that can affect human health. . . . Here is even more evidence for the need for an overhaul of our food safety system. A single food safety system anyone?"

CSPI (the Center for Science in the Public Interest) advised the USDA that new regulations must reduce the unacceptably high levels of Campylobacter and Salmonella in chicken and turkey.[36]

Several countries have placed tough import restrictions on U.S. poultry. India does not allow any poultry product into the country that has recorded an incident of avian influenza, which includes poultry from the United States.[37]

The Physicians Committee for Responsible Medicine (PCRM) found that 48 percent of all chicken products tested in a 2012 study were contaminated with E. coli. Even the outside of the plastic wrapping tested positive for E. coli.[38] The sampling was small and concentrated in 10 towns in southern California, but the group points out, "The numbers are what they are." E. coli is a bacterium often found in fecal matter. At one Ralph's supermarket location, five of six samples contained E. coli. Three contaminated samples dropped to the unacceptable range, according to USDA standards. One hundred percent of chicken samples tested positive at a Kroger store in Dallas. "I think most people don't know they are consuming fecal matter," said Susan Levin, a registered dietician and member of PCRM who advocates a vegan diet.[39] The group did not attempt to trace the contamination back to its source; it only wanted to show the numbers relating to pathogens found in study.

The Foodborne Diseases Active Surveillance Network, or FoodNet, is a CDC program that tracks foodborne infections. FoodNet has reported that since the period 1996–1999, the incidence of human Salmonella enteritidis (SE) infection has increased by 44 percent.[40] This change is mirrored in passive national surveillance data. The greatest relative increases were in young children, older adults, and FoodNet sites in the southern United States. Chicken and eggs get blamed for the major sources of infections.

The United States in 2013 took a giant step toward opening a big trade window with China. The USDA now allows China to export its own domestic chickens here, approving four Chinese poultry producing factories to ship only cooked poultry from birds raised in the United States.[41] Investigators trace much of our food contamination to imports. Things could get worse, considering China's dismal food safety record.

The USDA initiated a recall of contaminated poultry from Chile because the chicken tested positive for dioxin, a carcinogenic chemical. Later the recall was expanded to include all imports of poultry from Chile pending re-inspections. The United States is the ninth largest importer of Chilean agricultural products, according to the USDA.

"Globally, antimicrobial drug resistance is rapidly rising, with resultant increased illness and death. Of particular concern is Escherichia coli, the most common bacterium to cause invasive disease in humans," according to the NIH. "In Europe, increasing proportions of bloodstream infections caused by E. coli are resistant to third-generation cephalosporins. Resistant E. coli can be transmitted to humans from animals. A large proportion of resistant isolates causing human infections are derived from food animals.

However, lack of data has made it difficult to quantify the proportion of antimicrobial drug resistant E. coli infecting persons through food sources and the resultant effects on human health," according to the NIH.

The CDC published a detailed report in 2013 warning that the "improper use of antibiotics kills thousands and harms millions every year. Antibiotics used in food animals prevent, control, and treat disease, and promote the growth of the animals." But the CDC emphasizes that the routine use of antibiotics to promote growth is not necessary and should be phased out.

CSPI points out that one-third of the 12 resistant pathogens that the CDC considers a serious threat to Americans are found in food. "Antibiotic resistance is a health crisis that warrants attention: CDC estimates at least two million illnesses every year are from an antibiotic-resistant infection." CSPI cautions this may be understated as to the real public health burden.

Just as overuse of drugs in human medicine can lead to resistant bacteria, farm use can also promote resistance. In recent tests on ground turkey, the United States found that bacteria on meat from turkeys that were raised without antibiotics were resistant to fewer antibiotics than the bacteria found on turkeys that were raised with antibiotics.

A paper published in August 2013 on the CDC website states, "The number of avoidable deaths and the costs of health care potentially caused by third-generation cephalosporin use in food animals is staggering. Considering those factors, the ongoing use of these antimicrobial drugs in mass therapy and prophylaxis should be urgently examined and stopped, particularly in poultry, not only in Europe, but worldwide."[42]

Sliceable turkey meat was blamed for a 2002 eight-state outbreak of Listeriosis in the northeast United States. Seven people died, three stillbirths or miscarriages were reported, and 46 others became ill. The CDC says samples of turkey slices showed Listeria monocytogenes as the sources. The processing plant, operated by Pilgrim's Pride Foods in Franconia, Pennsylvania, recalled more than 27 million pounds of fresh and ready-to-eat frozen turkey and chicken products and voluntarily suspended operations.

The CDC warns, "Eating food contaminated with Listeria monocytogenes can result in Listeriosis, an uncommon but potentially fatal disease. The majority of Listeriosis cases occur among pregnant women, the elderly and persons with weakened immune systems. An illness in pregnant women can result in miscarriage, stillbirth or death of a newborn infant. Listeriosis often begins with influenza-like symptoms and sometimes with diarrhea, which might occur within one week after eating contaminated food. Symptoms might progress to include high fever, severe headache, and neck stiffness."[43]

The USDA's FSIS now requires its inspectors at poultry plants to begin sampling products for Salmonella and Campylobacter before shipment. If pathogens are discovered, the action establishes the prevalence of Salmonella in ground turkey at processing plants.

Meanwhile, China won't wait for more tests. In August 2013, China suspended imports of products from a Jennie-O turkey processing facility, according to the USDA.[44] Neither China nor the FSIS division of the U.S. Department of Agriculture offered an explanation. A spokesman for Hormel Foods, Jennie-O's parent company, told Meatingplace.com: "We are resolving a technical question with the Chinese and expect the matter to be cleared up in two to three weeks."

The 28-nation EU refuses to compromise with the United States on the chicken issue.[45] "US poultry producers have fewer sanitary demands on conditions for chicken, because once the chickens are slaughtered, they are dipped in a bleaching solution which kills all germs and bacteria," according to EUObserver.[46] The EU has banned imports of this kind of meat.

Chapter Five

Eggs

When many of us were growing up, it was safe to eat eggs. In fact, it was safe enough that we ate raw eggs mixed with chocolate icing our moms stirred in a bowl that would soon be licked clean by a little one hanging around the kitchen.

Enter Salmonella. It wasn't that long ago, the mid-1970s, when, almost simultaneously in many countries, Salmonella mysteriously began showing up in hens and their eggs. Federal food investigators discovered a strain of Salmonella enteritidis bacteria, known as SE.

Today, eggs top the list as the leading source of food poisoning in the United States. The CSPI says, "Hundreds, and possibly thousands, of people die every year from contaminated eggs."[1] Farms in the northeast United States produced the most tainted eggs. "With quick action back in the 1970s, the problem might have been stopped there. But the numerous federal agencies with oversight responsibilities for eggs didn't act. Instead, they competed with each other, stumbled over each other, and ultimately backed down in the face of industry pressure." Meanwhile, Salmonella enteritidis reached epidemic proportions.

In the summer of 1987, an outbreak of Salmonella-tainted eggs struck at Bird S. Coler Memorial Hospital in New York City, sickening 500 patients and staff.[2] Within two weeks, nine people had died from Salmonellosis. The contaminated eggs were traced to the Austin J. DeCoster egg operation, one of the country's biggest producers. Tainted eggs from his huge Hillandale Farms made headlines again, more than two decades later. A billion eggs were recalled after hundreds, perhaps thousands, of sicknesses were linked to the Salmonella-contaminated eggs. The FDA received criticism for failure to act in a timely manner.[3]

Illnesses from contaminated eggs increased five-fold through 1995, causing more than 200,000 to a million cases of Salmonella each year, according
to the CDC. The bacteria caused more reported deaths between 1988 and
1992 than any other foodborne pathogen, according to the CSPI.[4]

In 1990, the federal government agreed to draw up rules governing egg
farms. Representatives from consumer groups, egg farmers, and the USDA
finally came together on the same page on the issue. But nothing happened.
The USDA dropped the ball again.

Health officials, perhaps jumping the gun a bit, created a "runny egg rule"
in 1992 banning the practice of serving dishes with raw or undercooked eggs.
The rule did not set well with then Governor Jim Florio of New Jersey, who
staged a media event at a diner where he defiantly ordered eggs over easy as
TV cameras rolled.[5] And more than a few eyes rolled at news of the "runny
egg rule." Even late-night comedian Johnny Carson used the event for some
of his routines.

The responsibility of egg inspections today rests with the FDA. But similar to the required inspections of imported food and other products, our
government falls flat, with egg farm inspectors paying a visit to each farm on
the average of only once a decade.[6] The government also failed to initiate a
nationwide program, extremely successful in Pennsylvania, that, according
to the CSPI, "showed promise in reducing the number of food poisonings
from Salmonella enteritidis. However, federal support for that program was
discontinued in 1995, and no nationwide program has ever been implemented."[7]

Eggs look good after fecal material is removed and the shells are readied
to be placed in cardboard cartons and sent on their way to your neighborhood
grocery store for a personal examination by the consumer. But the FDA
performs a check only once every 10 years on the average for microbiological and chemical contaminations that are not visible to the naked eye.

The CSPI, in a presentation before the Senate Committee on Government
Affairs, presented a chronology of events that tells a huge and critically
important story titled "How a Tiny Foodborne Bacteria Outsmarted the Federal Government."[8]

- 1986—An outbreak sickens 3,000. CDC identifies eggs as the source of
  Salmonella food poisoning.
- 1987—USDA decides not to establish a mandatory Salmonella control
  program.
- 1989—Almost 8,500 Salmonella food poisonings are reported. USDA and
  FDA simultaneously develop competing Salmonella control programs.
- 1991—USDA begins a control program targeted only at flocks that have
  already been identified as the cause of human illness. Congress passes a
  law requiring egg refrigeration; USDA never enforces it.

- 1992—USDA and the Pennsylvania government begin a voluntary pilot control program.
- 1995—Congress cuts funding for successful pilot program at the request of the egg industry. More than 10,000 people are stricken with Salmonella food poisonings during the year.
- 2011—McDonald's begins looking for a new source for its popular Egg McMuffin breakfast item.[9] Target pulls its eggs off the shelves at about the same time the FDA is coming down hard on Sparboe Farms in Vincent, Iowa, the nation's fifth largest egg farm. Mercy for Animals, a consumer activist group, blows the whistle on the filth, unsanitary conditions, and repeated acts of animal cruelty, all captured on videotape via a hidden camera.[10]

The FDA cited serious violations at five different locations around the Sparboe plant site and 13 violations of a new rule adopted to prevent dangerous Salmonella outbreaks.[11] Mercy for Animals executive director Nathan Runkle told ABC News, "I saw workers do horrendous things to birds; they were thrown, grabbed by the neck, and slammed in and out of cages."[12]

A little more than a year later, Sparboe Farms was raided by dozens of federal Homeland Security agents and officers from U.S. Immigration and Customs Enforcement and Minnesota State Police.[13] Warnings issued to company officials contained details of violations of federal law, designed to help prevent Salmonella contaminations.

Another Salmonella outbreak in 2010 sickened thousands of people and resulted in a recall of 550 million contaminated eggs.[14] Salmonella, inside eggs laid by otherwise healthy hens, grows faster in temperatures above 45^0 F. It's estimated that almost five million eggs are contaminated with Salmonella each year.[15] "The elderly residents of nursing homes are especially at risk of death from Salmonella enteritis. Eighty-five percent of reported deaths from SE between 1988 and 1992 were from this group. Salmonella infections cause flu-like symptoms, such as diarrhea, abdominal pain, nausea, fever and chills, and can have more serious complications, such as rheumatoid arthritis, meningitis, kidney or heart disease, and death," according to the CSPI. Thorough cooking of eggs is the best way to kill the bacteria.

The much more dangerous Listeria monocytogenes can cause serious and sometimes fatal infections in young children, frail or elderly people, and others with weakened immune systems. Although healthy individuals may suffer only short-term symptoms such as high fever, severe headache, stiffness, nausea, abdominal pain, and diarrhea, Listeria infection can cause miscarriages and stillbirths among pregnant women.

While the FDA and the USDA work hard to compete with each other rather than cooperate to reach a common goal, once again we see that some countries are far ahead of the United States in critical food safety issues.

Sweden's aggressive Salmonella control program, in place since the mid-1980s, has prevented numerous outbreaks of Salmonella. [16] Only five flocks of hens and broilers have been identified as carrying Salmonella since 1987. Each bird is tested three times in its life. When flocks test positive for Salmonella, they are destroyed.

In the United States, 15 federal agencies and more than 70 interagency agreements vie for power and authority, competing against one another and causing fragmentation of responsibilities, major redundancies, and large gaps in enforcement. This causes a loss in both food safety and tax dollars.

The *Washington Post* in 2010 wrote: "Balkanization was a key factor in the government's failure to regulate eggs over the past two decades. [17] The push for federal rules on egg production stalled in the George H. W. Bush and Clinton administrations as the FDA and USDA dug into their own silos. It collapsed when the George W. Bush administration brought a renewed skepticism about regulation to the executive branch." [18]

Perhaps we should look across the pond for an answer to our issue with the egg. In the United States, federal law mandates that eggs be washed and sanitized before being packed in cartons and sold. [19] Those 28 countries making up the European Union, on the other hand, sell the Class A eggs, the best available, unwashed. It's the law in Europe that the eggs must not be washed. The EU has a reason for this . . . a very good reason. But to explain we must get a little personal with the hen.

Let's talk about her cuticle. She uses this coating around the egg to protect it against contamination before she lays the egg. This cuticle, or bloom, is designed to prevent moisture from forming on the egg and a carbon dioxide loss that would degrade the quality of the egg. This layer of natural coating from the hen, still wet when the egg emerges, dries within a few moments. This is an all-important barrier to bacterial ingress with an array of antimicrobial properties. Washing is prohibited because it would damage the cuticle, making eggs more susceptible to contamination from any pathogens rather than providing an additional safety zone. Yes, Mother Nature's way is the safe way.

Stroll through a supermarket in England and you'll see unrefrigerated eggs on shelves at room temperature. [20] Remember, it's the law in EU countries that eggs not be refrigerated before sale to the customers. Preventing condensation from forming also prevents the growth of bacteria on the shell that would likely permeate into the egg. Chilled eggs transported to your car and then to your home would cause the eggs to form the condensation that would lead to possible bacterial growth.

British egg farmers vaccinate hens against Salmonella, virtually eliminating the disease. The U.S. FDA reports nearly 150,000 illnesses each year from the consumption of eggs tainted with Salmonella. [21]

DHerbs.com points out that eating eggs can promote a host of diseases and pathologies: "Eggs can play a pivotal role in some female reproductive diseases including fibroid tumors, uterine cysts, breast cancer and tumors, and menstrual irregularities. Also, since these chicken eggs are sterilized or infertile, they are in fact impairing their own sexual fertility and potency."[22]

A 2012 study by the Stroke Prevention and Atherosclerosis Research Centre at Western University in Canada found that cholesterol in egg yolks is almost as dangerous as smoking cigarettes.[23] Carotid plaque area increased linearly after age 40 but increased exponentially with pack-years of smoking and with egg-yolk years, according to Dr. David Spence at Washington University. "What we have shown is that with aging, plaque builds up gradually in the arteries of Canadians, and egg yolks make it build up faster—about two-thirds as much as smoking. In the long haul, egg yolks are not okay for most Canadians," according to Dr. Spence.

Janice Stanger, PhD, who wrote *The Perfect Formula Diet: How to Lose Weight and Get Healthy Now With Six Kinds of Whole Foods*, wrote in her blog, "Chickens and eggs are interchangeable. An egg is a disassembled chick, since everything needed to form the baby bird is inside the egg. The shell forms a casing that allows the contents of the egg, under proper conditions, to rearrange themselves into a baby bird who will hatch and grow into a reproducing member of his or her species."[24] She goes on to say, "Chicks, whether assembled into birds or disassembled in eggs, are not an appetizing or health promoting food."

I found one of the best newspaper comments on the subject of contaminated eggs in a New Jersey *Star-Ledger* editorial board column, written after 500 million eggs were recalled from a filth-infested egg farm in 2010.[25] "Years ago, when Henny Penny was scratching out doomsday messages in the barnyard dirt, eggs were among the safest foods. But now they're produced in poultry mega-dormitories housing thousands. Just 192 egg companies own 95 percent of the nation's egg-laying hens, which means widespread contamination is more likely, if not inevitable."

They've become the incredible inedible eggs, and a recall of more than a half-billion has experts scrambling for an answer: Why can't the government better protect consumers? I think with the help of the EU, we may have answered that question.

Chapter Six

Beef and Pork

Here are just a few stories about bacteria in our beef:

- In 2009, Taiwan television produced a series of programs detailing what it called toxic U.S. beef exported to various countries around the world. "On January 1, 1989, the EU banned the import of U.S. beef produced with growth-promoting hormones. Since then, the EU and the US have been locked in a trade dispute that lasted for 20 years. The truth is, most toxic food in today's world are invented and produced by the US food industry in alliance with some profit-seeking scientists and a revenue-looking government," according to the program. [1]
- *Consumer Reports* conducted lab tests and found 3 to 7 percent of samples contained Listeria, Salmonella, or Staphylococcus aureus. [2] The study included samples of pork products from random stores across the country. Some of the bacteria found were resistant to multiple drugs or classes of drugs, according to the report. Yersinia enterocolitica was in 69 percent of the tested pork samples. It infects about 100,000 Americans a year, mostly children. [3]
- Four children died and nearly 700 other persons were infected in 1993 as a result of E. coli O157:H7 in undercooked hamburgers at Jack in the Box restaurants. [4] Significantly, this was the first deadly foodborne E. coli outbreak in the nation.
- "Since 1999, at least 343 people across the nation have been confirmed ill in foodborne illness outbreaks linked to Taco Bell," according to the Marler Clark law firm representing at least one victim of the Taco Bell Salmonella outbreak. [5]
- In 2007, a hamburger consumed by Stephanie Smith, a 22-year-old children's dance instructor in Minnesota, sent her into convulsions that grew

to the point doctors were forced to put her in a coma for nine weeks. When she awoke, her nervous system had been devastated and she was paralyzed. The hamburger, which her mother had cooked for her contained E. coli O157:H7.[6]

The Critical State of Antibiotics

We've overused antibiotics in cattle, pigs, and other meat animals for half a century, and now we humans are dearly paying the price. Eighty percent of the antibiotics used in the United States are for quickly fattening food animals. Bottom line? Antibiotic-resistant bacteria ends up in our food.

A 2013 study of meat products sampled from U.S. supermarkets found antibiotic-resistant bacteria in 81 percent of raw turkey, 69 percent of pork chops, 55 percent of ground beef, and 39 percent of raw chicken breasts, wings, and thighs.[7]

The U.S. FDA's National Antimicrobial Resistance Monitoring System (NARMS) conducted the project. The release of the project results on February 5, 2013, drew little attention from the national news media.

Antibiotic, or antimicrobial, resistance is simply drug resistance caused largely by the increasing subtherapeutic and therapeutic use of antibiotics in food animals, a growing problem in the United States. Using antibiotics to treat sick animals is not the real culprit, however. The subtherapeutic use of antibiotics as a preventative measure against illness in animals has seemingly had the opposite effect. Rather than preventing illness, the use of smaller levels of antibiotics has just trained bacteria to resist their enemies, making them stronger. These bacteria may then infect human populations, making treatment more difficult. According to the FDA and the Animal Health Institute, pharmaceutical makers in 2011 sold nearly 30 million pounds of antibiotics to be fed to domestic food-producing animals.

The FDA obligingly offers the entire NARMS report without cost to the public but advises that it is "approximately 11 megabytes and takes between 8–11 minutes to download a one megabyte file using the average dial up internet connection." Was the FDA discouraging us to see the full report? Perhaps. But, if you take the time and search deep enough, you'll find the report is broken down in summary form.

The increased amounts of antibiotics fed to hogs and cattle have jumped to critically dangerous proportions across the country. Leading scientists, addressing 120 U.S. congressional staff members and others in March 2012, presented evidence that when antibiotics are given inappropriately to cattle, swine, and poultry, we promote the growth of new strains of bacteria resistant to existing antibiotics, and the result can infect humans. The new bacteria pose a potentially fatal risk for us.

In early 2012, Congresswoman Louise Slaughter (D-NY), the only micro-biologist in Congress, blames the FDA's lack of strong action on the problem, adding, "This fight is probably the fight of a lifetime."[8] The FDA responded by issuing a voluntary initiative suggesting antibiotics not be used for so-called production purposes. By law, the FDA has the authority and responsibility to protect public health, not the animal producers.

Back in 2012, the FDA announced that it was taking steps to protect public health and promote the judicious use of medically important antibiotics in food-producing animals. "It is critical that we take action to protect public health," said FDA commissioner Margaret A. Hamburg, MD.[9] "The new strategy will ensure farmers and veterinarians care for animals while ensuring the medicines people need remain safe and effective. We are also reaching out to animal producers who operate on a smaller scale or in remote locations to help ensure the drugs they need to protect the health of their animals are still available."

Food safety watchdogs warned that the FDA's new policies that were intended to reduce the overuse of important antibiotics in animal production are tragically flawed. "They rely too heavily on the drug industry and animal producers to act voluntarily in the best interest of consumers. Protecting public health is an authority and a responsibility that rests squarely with the FDA," according to Food Safety Director Caroline Smith DeWaal of the CDC.[10]

Ms. DeWall points to what she describes as decades of misuse that led to some common pathogens like Salmonella becoming more virulent and less treatable. "The FDA knows it can no longer afford to ignore antibiotic resistance. In March 2012, the agency took a step in the right direction by banning certain extra-label uses of cephalosporin in certain food-producing animals," she said.[11]

One final statement from the CSPI director: "The problem of antimicrobial resistance, and the contribution of animal agriculture to that problem, is urgent and global. The United States needs to take a leadership role in bringing comprehensive, effective action, in both the agricultural and medical spheres, to bear. The time for half-measures and voluntary steps has passed."[12]

Mad Cow Disease

The U.S. beef industry's problems continue. Indonesia banned imports of beef from the United States in June 2013 after the unexpected discovery of a new case of mad cow disease in California. Scientists say the cow did not acquire the disease from eating feed, and no other cattle were affected. This marked the first case of mad cow disease since 2006. Indonesia supplemented its beef import by ordering more of its meat from Australia and Canada.

Ractopamine

Could 160 countries be wrong in banning U.S.-grown and U.S.-produced beef because of one drug?[13] Ractopamine, a beta agonist drug used on pigs, cattle, and turkeys, increases weight gain and builds muscles in the animals and sickens or kills more pigs than any other livestock drug. The FDA admits in a Freedom of Information document that it was forced to submit to the media that more than 160,000 pigs were reported to have suffered ill effects since Ractopamine hit the market. Pigs suffered from hyperactivity, trembling, broken limbs, inability to walk, and death.

Ractopamine caused a stir after the 1999 FDA's approval of the drug for use on food animals. The issue caused a trade disagreement between the United States and Taiwan that has zero tolerance for the drug in pork and beef. It's no wonder the governments of more than 160 countries including Russia and China express serious doubts about the drug to the extent of banning it altogether.

More doubts surfaced in the United States when it was discovered that the FDA's approval of Ractopamine was based on tests conducted by Elanco, the company that produces the drug.[14] No wonder scores of countries doubt the safety of Ractopamine. Another reason points to the lack of support with the data provided by Elanco. The tests raised more questions about the safety of the drug in that "only one human study was used in the safety assessment by Elanco and among the six healthy young men who participated, one man was removed from the test because his heart began racing and pounding abnormally," according to the report.[15]

The Russian publication *Pravda* reported, "Ractopamine affects the human cardiovascular system, and in some cases can cause food poisoning."[16] The article quoted unnamed sources without providing any backup research. *Pravda* added that Russia was the fourth largest importer of U.S. meat and spent about $500 million a year on the imported meat. The Russian market consumed 0.6 percent of all beef and 1.4 percent of pork produced in the United States.[17]

The United States regards the ban of meat imports as a political move. According to American analysts, Russia has reacted to the adoption of the Magnitsky Act by the U.S. Congress.[18] On December 6, the U.S. Senate almost unanimously (92–4) approved the bill that imposed visa and financial sanctions against Russian officials involved in the death of Sergei Magnitsky, a lawyer of the Hermitage investment fund. The first three parts of this document are devoted to the interaction of Russia and the United States in the WTO. In particular, the bill abolishes the Jackson-Vanik amendment for Russia and Moldova, which was adopted in 1974, according to *Pravda*.

Now proponents of the drug, specifically the U.S. government, have found a work-around to get by with a smaller amount of Ractopamine in meat that might satisfy at least some of the other 160 countries. The United States wants the Codex Alimentarius Commission to set a standard residue level for Ractopamine in meat.[19] The United States pressured the commission until the summer of 2012 when the Codex vote of 69–67 set a 10 parts-per-billion limit for Ractopamine in beef and pork. Much to the consternation of U.S. officials, the European Food Safety Authority has ruled that there is little or no evidence to suggest that any level of Ractopamine is safe.

Since the approval of the drug, the U.S. FDA's Veterinary Medicine division has fielded more than 200,000 reports of adverse side effects in pigs fed Ractopamine, ranging from lameness to hyperactivity.[20] Many American food companies such as Chipotle and Whole Foods Market also refuse to sell meat that has been exposed to the growth stimulant.[21]

Several major countries including Canada, Brazil, Mexico, Japan, and South Korea in addition to the United States consider Ractopamine safe. But following the Codex Alimentarius vote action, the European Union reaffirmed its position that an international standard for Ractopamine is not justified.[22] The EU statement also warned that there is insufficient data upon which to make a proposal for maximum residue limits (MRLs) for Ractopamine and that risks to human health cannot be ruled out.[23]

Zilpaterol

In addition to Ractopamine, at least one more animal drug is at issue. South Korea in 2013 discovered that more than 75 tons of U.S. beef had been counterfeited to make it appear that it had originated in other countries. Importers in South Korea had bypassed tough restrictions on U.S. beef that contained a banned additive, Zilpaterol, a growth promoter.[24] Taiwan strictly prohibits Zilpaterol in food products.[25] The U.S. Department of Agriculture in 2006 approved this highly toxic chemical for use in cattle in Mexico and South Africa but not in the United States or other countries.

The U.S. FDA lists Zilpaterol as a Type B Medicated Feed supplement for increased rate of weight gain in cattle. Several Asian nations like China and many European countries have not approved Zilpaterol for use in meat.[26] Use of the additive produced some negative side effects. This report came a couple of years after South Korea suspended U.S. beef imports out of fears of also importing mad cow disease. The demand for the U.S. beef containing Zilpaterol is simple economics. It's 25–30 percent cheaper, providing restaurants a boost in the bottom line by simply changing the label on the meat.

Hormone-Fed Beef

VegNews, a premier vegan lifestyle magazine, reminds its readers that with the rejection of Ractopamine in many countries this is not the first time that

American animal products have been banned on the grounds of public safety.[27] The EU prohibits hormone-fed beef. U.S. trading partners such as Japan have outlawed the synthetically produced hormone bovine somatotropin (artificial bovine somatotropin is made by using recombinant DNA technology and is called recombinant bovine growth hormone, or rBGH) in dairy cattle, but it is commonly used in America to increase milk production.[28] Here's the problem: bovine somatotropin skews hormone levels in consumers that can lead to prostate and breast cancers. The American Cancer Society addresses the problem but leaves us with more questions than answers.[29] "Concerns about possible health effects on humans from milk produced using rBGH have focused on 2 main issues," the American Cancer Society reports.

"First, does drinking milk from rBGH-treated cows increase blood levels of growth hormone or IGF-1 in consumers? If it does, would this be expected to have any health effects in people, including increasing the risk of cancer? Several scientific reviews have looked at these issues and are the main focus of this document.

"Second, cows treated with rBGH tend to develop more udder infections (mastitis). These cows are given more antibiotics than cows not given rBGH. Does this increased use of antibiotics lead to more antibiotic-resistant bacteria, and is this a health concern for people?" This remains a concern, but it has not been fully examined in humans, according to the American Cancer Society.[30]

The Other White Meat

Pork, the "other white meat," is a good example of what's in our meat. *Consumer Reports* magazine conducted a scientific and detailed study and sampling from 40 brands of pork products from across the country. The results showed 69 percent of the pork chops and ground pork sampled tested positive for Yersinia enterocolitica, a bacteria that can cause abdominal pain, fever, diarrhea, joint pain, and skin rash.

Inspections

By 2014, U.S. inspections of slaughterhouses and other meat processing plants continued to come up short with sparse, ineffective, and near nonexistent guarantees of strict enforcement. During a four-year investigation, inspectors noted nearly 45,000 violations, including fecal matter on carcasses and repeat serious violators who were allowed to continue operations. Inspectors ordered suspensions of operations only a couple dozen times.

The Office of the Inspector General for the USDA opened an investigation of food safety and inspections at swine slaughter plants.[31] Eight out of the 30 plants visited during the OIG inspections revealed that the inspectors at the plants did not always examine the internal organs of carcasses as required or failed to take enforcement actions against plants in violation. The OIG says this amounts to a reduced assurance that inspectors are effectively identifying meat that should not enter the food supply. In a review of 158 humane handling violations issued to the 30 plants, the USDA found 10 instances of egregious violations where inspectors did not issue suspensions. As a result, the plants did not improve their slaughter practices, according to the Inspector General's report.

The USDA says 8,600 federal meat inspectors currently work in 6,300 processing and packing plants in the United States. The practice of hiding vital food safety facts from the public spreads wider and faster every month. In British Columbia, quite amazingly, the Agriculture Minister says that keeping secret any information about farm disease outbreaks will better protect the public.[32]

Food safety experts agree that standards for safe beef in the United States are lower than those in Europe and in several other countries including Japan.

INHUMANE TREATMENT OF FOOD ANIMALS

Now that we have our cattle and pigs filled with antibiotics, hormones, and feed inundated with a variety of chemicals, they are fat, happy, and ready for a trip. The last few inhumane steps in the lives of thousands of animals is appalling and hideous, filled with gruesome stories of atrocious beating, prodding, and dragging animals nearly dead to slaughterhouses.

The full story has to be publicized if these horrific acts are to be stopped. A video produced by a whistleblower vividly shows slaughterhouse workers bulldozing sick "downer cows," pushing them in for processing and eventual public consumption.[33] The video, released by the Humane Society of the United States, shows workers using repeated electric shocks on cows too weak to stand. Inspectors failed to vigorously enforce the numbers of violations of the Humane Methods of Slaughter Act, posing major health problems for consumers.

Publicity surrounding the treatment of the sick cows helped to prompt the largest recall of beef in the history of the United States: 143 million pounds, an entire two-year output of beef. On the heels of the revelation of what was going on in beef processing plants, several states rushed to protect big business, passing "ag-gag" laws and prohibiting any video recording in any slaughterhouse.[34] Instead of stopping the inhumane practices, lawmakers in several states, in effect, allowed the violations to continue, but in secret.

Another video surfaced in May 2012 documenting animal cruelty by a pork supplier in Wyoming.[35] The nationally seen video shows "downer" cows, unable to walk and barely able to move, being violently pushed with a forklift and repeatedly prodded, and dragged to slaughter.[36] The plant, Westland/Hallmark Meat Co., closed its doors, was sued by the U.S. government, and later was assessed a fine of $300,000, the largest animal-abuse case judgment in U.S history. However, Westland/Hallmark Meat was broke, and the fine was never paid.

Members of the Humane Society of the United States filed a lawsuit against Smithfield Foods, the processor that supplies the pork to McDonald's, alleging that Smithfield maintains its pigs in deplorable conditions.[37] The Humane Society conducted an in-depth investigation and found "animals had bitten their bars so incessantly that blood from their mouths coated the fronts of their crates. The breeding pigs also suffered injuries from sharp crate protrusions and open pressure sores that developed from their unyielding confinement. Three times, the investigator informed employees that a pig was thrown into a dumpster alive. The animal had been shot in the forehead with a captive bolt gun, which is designed to render an animal unconscious, and was thrown in the dumpster still alive and breathing."[38]

The investigative report included a quote from the CEO of the Humane Society, Wayne Pacelle: "If this is the best that Smithfield can do, it is evident that there are terrible problems in the nation's pig industry. It is indefensible for Smithfield to allow its sows to linger in crates barely larger than their bodies for months on end."[39]

Now, the meat industry continues pushing for ag-gag laws that prohibit any pictures being made at meat processing plants or slaughterhouses. In other words, "we don't want the public to see our dirty deeds that we're doing." The measures being introduced in several state houses would prevent citizens from documenting animal abuses in the plants. Only Iowa, Kansas, Missouri, Montana, North Dakota, and Utah have adopted ag-gag laws since 1990.

Good news comes from Governor Bill Haslam, a republican from Tennessee, who vetoed an ag-gag bill reaching his desk, saying the bill's provisions are "constitutionally suspect" with regard to the First Amendment to the U.S. Constitution.[40] This is a major victory in a fight against agricultural conglomerates and support corporations.

The movement against the abuse has attracted the support of not only the Humane Society of the United States, but others as well, such as singers Emmylou Harris and Carrie Underwood and comedienne Ellen DeGeneres.[41] Ag-gag laws have been introduced in more than a dozen states.[42] Newspaper editorials in the *New York Times* and the *Boston Globe* along with small and large newspapers in California, Connecticut, Indiana, North Carolina, Pennsylvania, and Tennessee oppose the anti-whistleblower bills.[43,44] Hopefully, Congress first will direct the USDA to strictly enforce applicable laws already on the books and direct U.S. attorneys throughout the nation to vigorously prosecute violators to the limits of the law.

All this secrecy in slaughterhouses doesn't faze some of our neighbors to the north. If the idea gets off the ground, you may not want to eat steak in Canada. Its conservative government wants to give meat processors the authority to process the carcasses of already dead animals. Strong opposition comes from the New Democrats in Canada.[45]

The McRib and Azodicarbonamide

Picture this: a compound so potentially dangerous that it is banned throughout Europe and Australia. Singapore's tough laws against the use of the additive azodicarbonamide include fines up to $450,000 and 15 years in prison.[46] "It's a respiratory sensitizer that potentially contributes to asthma through occupational exposure," England's Health and Safety Agent said in the *Time Magazine* article, "Why Lovin' the McRib Isn't Heart Smart."[47] The United States limits azodicarbonamide to 45 parts per million in commercial flour products, based on analysis of lab testing. The additive can also be found in many rubbery products such as floor mats and gym shoes, products in the photography and electronics industries, and a wide range of polymers, including polyvinyl chloride, polyolefins, and natural and synthetic rubbers.

Azodicarbonamide helps to make up a complex but tasty menu item at the world's largest fast-food restaurant chain.[48] You won't see meat falling off the bone of McDonald's McRib because it isn't a rib and it doesn't have a bone. More accurately, it's only a meat by-product. Azodicarbonamide along with polysorbate, 80 ammonium sulfate, and 67 other ingredients make up the McRib. Want to know more? Some of those ingredients include "a mixture of tripe, heart, and scalded stomach," according to the developer of the restructured meat product from which the McRib is made.[49] He's Richard Mandigo, a professor from the University of Nebraska, quoted in a 1995 article in *Chicago Magazine*. "The comminuted meat mixture is mixed with salt and water to extract salt-soluble proteins. These extracted proteins are critical to produce a 'glue,' which binds muscle pieces together. These muscle pieces may then be reformed to produce a 'meat log' of specific form or shape. The log is then cut into steaks or chops which, when cooked, are similar in appearance and texture to their intact muscle counterparts," according to the article.

"Most people would be extremely unhappy if they were served heart or tongue on a plate," Mandigo observed. "But flaked into a restructured product it loses its identity."

Pathogens from Tenderizing

Meat tenderizing takes place in your home, at butcher shops, and in major meat processing facilities. One process, with a little-publicized food safety issue, involves penetrating the meat with blades, pins, needles, or any mechanical device. It tenderizes the meat but drives any pathogen deep into it, resulting in a need for more than normal increased temperatures to kill the buried pathogen.

In 2003, the CDC determined that blade-tenderized injections into meat resulted in 13 persons becoming ill, and half of them had to be hospitalized. The process is often referred to as "blading" or "needling."[50]

In late 2012, the *Kansas City Star* published a revealing investigation titled "Beef's Raw Edges, Building Bigger Cattle: An Industry Overdose."[51] Reporter Mike McGraw's research delved into the industry's increased reliance on mechanical tenderization of meat "exposing Americans to a higher risk of E. coli poisoning." Most of the industry resists labeling such products. I found one exception. Mechanically tenderized beef sold at Costco clearly labels that the meat is "blade tenderized."

The *Star*, using the federal Freedom of Information Act, obtained inspection records for the most recent two-year period at the four largest beef slaughter plants. Here is one example of an inspector's notes: "Massive fecal contamination; multiple carcasses with varying degrees of fecal contamination; periods of very significant fecal, ingesta and abscess contamination."[52]

The *Kansas City Star* also reported that a medium-rare steak, consumed at an Applebee's restaurant by Margaret Lamkin, age 87, resulted in sickness that led to her colon being destroyed and leaving her to wear a colostomy bag for the rest of her life.[53] Ms. Lamkin, like all of us, had no idea she had eaten a steak that had been run through a mechanical tenderizer. She said in documents filed with her lawsuit that the contaminated meat came from National Steak Processors Inc., which claimed it got the steak from a U.S. plant run by Brazilian-based JBS, the largest beef packer in the world.

The newspaper concluded that the mechanical process "exposes Americans to a higher risk of E.coli poisoning than cuts of meat that have not been tenderized."

The USDA reports that between 2003 and 2009, 174 illnesses, including one death, were traced to mechanically tenderized beef. E. coli O157:H7 was the culprit. The tenderizing process drives any bacteria on the surface deep into the center of the meat. When the meat is cooked rare or medium rare, the chance of pathogen contamination increases.[54]

LOOKING AHEAD

The Philippines strictly enforces some of the toughest food safety laws in the world. The country touts its sanitary and phytosanitary measures that it imposes on all imports entering the country.[55] Even the pest risk assessment conducted by the Philippines Department of Agriculture for fresh vegetables and fruits is among the most thorough in the world.

Do U.S. food safety officials try to emulate the high standards in the Philippines or applaud their efforts to hold foodborne illnesses at a minimum? Not a chance. Instead, the Philippines food safety standards remain a thorny issue for the United States, which has vowed to oppose them because they block its access to the country's markets, according to the U.S. Trade Representative (USTR).[56] Once again, here are all the appearances of our government looking out for big business above safeguarding the health of the consumer.

The USTR website states that the Philippines sanitary policies "impede" the entry of U.S. exports. The Philippines "imposes very high standards on the handling of frozen meat, which is primarily imported, that do not apply to the handling of freshly slaughtered meat, which is exclusively domestic."

The Philippines government's tough food safety rules, regulations, and laws should be implemented by the U.S. government's food safety agencies.

In the future, don't be surprised to see a hamburger produced from 10,000 stem cells extracted from cattle, left to multiply by more than a billion times. Muscle tissue will be used to formulate the burgers in vitro. Dr. Mark Post of Maastricht University, ranked as one of the best schools in the Netherlands in 2011, and his team of Dutch researchers predict even steaks and chops could be formulated in the future.[57] News of test tube meat will likely set off another round of media stories similar to tales about "pink slime" but much, much worse.

Chapter Seven

Milk

Julie Riggs lived in a small town in Missouri and decided raw goat milk would benefit both her husband and her nine-year-old daughter.[1] Instead, they ended up in the hospital after drinking E. coli–tainted unpasteurized goat milk. The condition of Ms. Riggs's daughter grew critical. Her pancreas shut down. Dialysis began, constant vomiting continued, blood transfusions were administered, and insulin was injected. Ms. Riggs, living in her daughter's hospital room for many weeks, feared seizures or strokes might be next. "I could have lost either one of them," she said.[2] But after a month in the hospital, she and her daughter went home, although her daughter continued to have stomachaches and pains. Her daughter and husband soon recovered fully. "The risk of drinking unpasteurized milk is not worthy of anything I can think of," Ms. Riggs said.[3]

Kalee Prue lived in Connecticut and had been convinced that drinking raw milk was a healthy choice.[4] After drinking unpasteurized milk, however, she became ill and tested positive for E. coli contamination from consuming the raw milk. Her kidneys began shutting down, prompting almost continuous dialysis and 20 treatments of plasmapheresis. After 33 days in the hospital and plasma units from 400 different people, she was recovering.

Mary McGonigle-Martin was living in California when a dairy farmer told her that his unpasteurized milk had been tested and was safe.[5] She later said she had been lulled into a "false sense of security." Her seven-year-old son became infected after contracting E. coli and soon was hooked to a ventilator and dialysis was started. "I thought he would die any moment," she said.[6] It was only after three years of treatments that she could say life was back to normal.

The CDC provided these interviews it conducted with some of the patients and their families to give us all a better understanding of the dangers in consuming unpasteurized milk or foods made with raw milk. The CDC warns that a person consuming raw milk can develop severe or even life-threatening diseases, such as Guillain-Barré syndrome, which can cause paralysis, and hemolytic uremic syndrome, which can result in kidney failure and stroke.[7]

One hundred years ago, 48 people died and 1,400 others were infected in the Boston area from drinking contaminated unpasteurized milk, often referred to as raw milk. The unpasteurized milk issue had been discussed in medical journals prior to the infections, but only on a limited basis. Today, California law requires a lengthy warning label on raw milk containers, advising: "WARNING: Raw (unpasteurized) milk and raw milk dairy products may contain disease-causing micro-organisms. Persons at highest risk of disease from these organisms include newborns and infants; the elderly; pregnant women; those taking corticosteroids, antibiotics or antacids; and those having chronic illnesses or other conditions that weaken their immunity."[8] Nothing could be clearer regarding the extreme dangers of consuming raw milk.

In fact, that should be enough to make most people turn and look for the pasteurized milk in their supermarket's dairy section. The CDC reported that between 1993 and 2006, unpasteurized products caused a disproportionate number of outbreaks, 150 times more than outbreaks linked to pasteurized milk.[9] The report also states, "Numerous pathogens can contaminate dairy products and cause illness and death." Pasteurization eliminates those pathogens.

Drinking raw milk sickened more than 100 people in Pennsylvania in 2012, the largest such outbreak in that state's history.[10] Unpasteurized milk from Your Family Cow dairy in Chambersburg, Pennsylvania, contained the pathogen Campylobacter, according to the CDC.[11] Health officials say the dairy obtained the necessary permit and passed inspections prior to the outbreak.[12] This demonstrates the ongoing hazards of unpasteurized milk in that there is one step that must be taken with raw milk and that is pasteurization. The Your Family Cow dairy incident marked the fifth outbreak of 2012 from drinking raw milk.[13]

It's true that fewer people are poisoned by pathogens in raw milk than those who might get sick from Salmonella in produce. But, there are far fewer people drinking raw (unpasteurized) milk. It's important enough to repeat: The rate of food-poisoning outbreaks caused by unpasteurized or raw milk and dairy products is 150 times greater than outbreaks linked to pasteurized milk, according to new research.

LiveScience, a daily report on health issues, quotes food safety professor Douglas Powell from Kansas State University: "Raw milk is riskier than most foods."[14] While certainly a larger number of people get sick yearly from eating tainted tomatoes or lettuce, there are many more consumers of those foods than raw milk, he said. Bacteria commonly found in the digestive tracts of farm animals, including Campylobacter and E. coli O157, can easily find their way into milk as it is pumped and bottled on a farm, according to Powell.[15]

"Fecal matter just ends up in the milk—it's not like you can see it," he said. "No inspectors can see it—this isn't CSI, where the bacteria just magically line up." Children comprised nearly a third of those sickened in the 2012 Chambersburg outbreak, according to the report. Children, pregnant women, and people with compromised immune systems are at high risk for complications from Campylobacter infections. "As adults, you're free to choose," Powell said. "But don't give it to our kids."

Consumers can never be certain that unpasteurized milk is free of pathogens. You can have it tested, certified, and retested, but the safest route to take is simply not to drink it.

Raw milk can contain dangerous bacteria, including Listeria, Staphylococcus, E. coli, Campylobacter, Yersinia, Coxiella, and Brucella.[16] Federal law prohibits the interstate shipment of raw milk and cheese made from raw milk. Some states allow the sale of unpasteurized milk within their borders. I hear the argument anytime the subject of raw milk comes up that pasteurization kills "good" bacteria. The point is that the bacterium that is destroyed during pasteurization realistically saves lives.

A 2012 outbreak of E. coli infections linked to raw milk consumption sickened 19 people in Oregon, including four children who were hospitalized.[17] The Oregon Health Authority reported that 15 of the 19 cases were children under 19 years of age. All of those stricken were confirmed to have consumed unpasteurized milk from Foundation Farm in Oregon.[18] Hemolytic uremic syndrome (HUS), a type of kidney failure, developed in the four children ranging in age from one to 13.[19] The problem with treatment is that physicians cannot use antibiotics that could heighten the possibility of kidney failure.

In the same year, an E.coli outbreak in Missouri sickened 12 people in six counties.[20] All had been confirmed as having consumed raw (unpasteurized) milk. The Missouri Department of Health and Senior Services (MDHSS) warned that the risk in drinking unpasteurized milk "is comparable to that of eating raw ground beef or raw ground poultry and, in many cases, the germs that are present are similar. The most common germs found in raw milk include Listeria monocytogenes, Salmonella spp., Campylobacter jejuni, Yersinia enterocolitica, Escherichia coli (E. coli O157-H7), and mastitis-causing germs such as Streptococcus aureus. Some of these are found in the environment and/or in the feces of animals commonly used for milk. Germs may vary according to the time of year, geographic location, herd size, and farm management practices."[21,22]

In 1985, an outbreak of Salmonellosis infected 16,284 people and killed at least two others. Federal health officials identified the source as Salmonella typhimurium–contaminated milk from the Hillfarm dairy in Melrose Park, Illinois.[23] All but 1,059 of the victims were from Illinois. The organism "directly caused the deaths of two people and was a factor in the deaths of four others," according to the Illinois Department of Public Health.[24]

The *St. Louis Post-Dispatch* reported in April 2012, "Raw milk enthusiasts say an E. coli outbreak in Missouri won't change their preference for unpasteurized dairy products. MooGrass Farms near Collinsville sells about 200 gallons of raw cow, goat and sheep milk each week, mostly to families from the St. Louis area, said the farm's manager, Kevin Kosiek. His customers appreciate the taste of whole raw milk as well as the lack of heat processing that kills some of the nutrients."[25]

"This is not a fad," Kosiek said. "People are going back to where people used to get their food, and that's farmers doing natural, organic things."[26]

It's estimated that less than 1 percent of the milk consumed in the United States is raw, although its popularity is growing. The CDC has some attention-getting facts about consumption of unpasteurized milk: From 1998 through 2011, the CDC reported 148 outbreaks due to consumption of raw milk or raw milk products. The food poisonings resulted in 2,384 illnesses, 284 hospitalizations, and two deaths. Escherichia coli, Campylobacter, Salmonella, or Listeria caused most of these illnesses.

A study released by the CDC in February 2012 examined the number of dairy outbreaks in the United States during a 13-year period. Between 1993 and 2006, 60 percent (73/121) of dairy-related outbreaks reported to the CDC were linked to raw milk products. Three-quarters of these outbreaks occurred in states where the sale of raw milk was legal at the time. Experts also found that those sickened in raw milk outbreaks were 13 times more likely to be hospitalized than those who got ill from pasteurized milk during an outbreak.

As I mentioned previously, federal law does not allow the sale of unpasteurized milk in interstate commerce. It's up to each state to draw up specific laws regarding raw milk, leaving the question in more or less a hodgepodge.

States that allow the legal sale of raw milk for human consumption have more raw milk–related outbreaks of illness than states that do not allow raw milk to be sold legally, according to the CDC.[27] Raw milk sales are illegal in Nevada, Louisiana, Montana, Iowa, West Virginia, New Jersey, and Maryland. Other states allow retail sales or farm sales or both. The sale of raw milk to consumers is prohibited in Canada.

According to the analysis by the CDC between 1993 and 2006, more than 1,500 people in the United States became sick from drinking raw milk or eating cheese made from raw milk.[28] But keep in mind, as with other foodborne disease outbreaks, only a small percentage of those actually sickened are reported. A raw milk consumption study in Minnesota, released in late

2013, confirmed the public's reporting of foodborne diseases.[29] "The number of illnesses ascertained as part of documented outbreaks likely represents a small portion of the actual number of illnesses associated with this food product," the study concluded.

After studying the issue, one of the clearest facts I saw was this: Pasteurization was invented in 1864 and was beginning to be used in the United States in the 1890s. When pasteurization became the norm after the turn of the century, around the early 1900s, the number of deaths from illnesses like bovine tuberculosis, easily transmitted to humans through raw milk, plummeted.

Yes, unpasteurized milk is a killer.

Chapter Eight

Seafood

How unsafe is the seafood we consume? I'll gently give you the bad news: We import 91 percent of the seafood we eat. We inspect only 2 percent of the seafood we eat.[1]

I know, that was not too gentle. But it will take some kick-in-the-doors, ask-questions-later type actions to force a revelatory sign from Congress and the White House that they care about this potentially deadly problem. Our watchdog government agency, charged by law with the duty and responsibility to make sure our food is safe, fails us miserably on the hundreds of docks and other ports of entry around the nation.

Look at the European Union, where 50 percent of its imported seafood receives the inspectors' stamps of approval or it's rejected.[2]

It's difficult to imagine the major shortage of inspectors in the United States. For example, in 2010 the FDA had only 92 full-time border inspectors.[3] Each inspector's job description consisted of checking 56 million pounds of seafood, physically examining samples of shipments, testing the seafood for a variety of deadly pathogens, and scanning for toxic contaminants. Additionally, inspectors are required to inspect processing facilities at the origin of the shipments, which is not being done. Lack of proper funding means fewer inspectors, resulting in the federally mandated responsibilities being bypassed. Inspectors accomplish little of what's required.

Tainted imports, lack of inspections, and increased consumption of the products increase food safety dangers as they relate to seafood. The average American now eats about 17 pounds of seafood a year compared with about 10 pounds during the 1980s. As we eat more seafood, we encounter more marine toxins, chemicals, heavy metals, bacteria, and parasites.

Around the World

China leads the world in aquaculture, followed by India, Indonesia, Bangladesh, Norway, and Chile. The United States is 13th in the aquaculture world.[4]

Here's where we get our seafood:

- Shrimp from Asian countries and Ecuador
- Atlantic salmon from Canada, Norway, and Chile
- Tilapia from China
- Scallops from China and some from Canada, Mexico, and Japan[5]

Diseases

The most common diseases caused by marine toxins in the United States in order of incidence are scombrotoxic fish poisoning, ciguatera poisoning, paralytic shellfish poisoning, neurotoxic shellfish poisoning, and amnesic shellfish poisoning, according to the CDC.[6]

Scombrotoxic fish poisoning, also known as scombroid or histamine fish poisoning, is caused by bacterial spoilage of certain finfish such as tuna, mackerel, bonito, and, rarely, other fish. Ciguatera poisoning, or ciguatera, is caused by eating contaminated tropical reef fish. Ciguatoxins that cause ciguatera poisoning are actually produced by microscopic sea plants called dinoflagellates.

Paralytic shellfish poisoning is caused by a different dinoflagellate with a different toxin than that causing ciguatera poisoning.[7] These dinoflagellates have a red-brown color and can grow to such numbers that they cause red streaks to appear in the ocean called "red tides." This toxin is known to concentrate within certain shellfish that typically live in the colder coastal waters of the Pacific states and New England, though the syndrome has been reported in Central America, according to the CDC.[8]

Amnesic shellfish poisoning is a rare syndrome caused by a toxin made by a microscopic, red-brown, saltwater plant, a diatom called Nitzchia pungens. The toxin produced by this diatom is concentrated in shellfish such as mussels and causes disease when the contaminated shellfish are eaten.

The Center for Science in the Public Interest continually studies all phases of foodborne illnesses and says seafood by far is the most hazardous to eat, followed by poultry, eggs, and beef. The number of illnesses from pathogens contracted in consuming seafood is almost three times greater than that contracted by eating poultry.

The CDC has a matter-of-fact warning about the dangers of eating these fish.[9] Histidine, one of the essential amino acids, "will convert to histamine by bacterial overgrowth in fish that has been improperly stored after capture.

Histamine and other scombrotoxins are resistant to cooking, smoking, canning, or freezing. Fish contaminated with histamine may possess a peppery, sharp, salty, or 'bubbly' feel but may also look, smell, and taste normal. The key to prevention is to make sure that the fish is properly iced, refrigerated, or immediately frozen after it is caught."[10]

More than 50,000 cases of ciguatera poisonings occur globally every year. The risk to travelers to some of the high endemic areas is estimated as high as 3 in 100 people. Geographical areas of risk include the Canary Islands, the eastern Mediterranean, and the western Gulf of Mexico, according to the CDC. Carriers of the pathogen are barracuda, grouper, moray eel, sea bass or sturgeon, and amberjack. Ciguatera fish poisoning occurs after eating reef fish contaminated with toxins such as ciguatoxin or maitotoxin. These potent toxins originate from small marine organisms (dinoflagellates) that grow on and around coral reefs.

The toxins concentrate as they pass up the food chain to large carnivorous fish (usually larger than 6 lb, 2.7 kg) and finally to humans. Toxins concentrate in fish liver, intestines, roe, and head, according to the CDC.[11]

This may come as a surprise to you: Eating finfish causes about 50 percent more outbreaks and illnesses than shellfish consumption. That doesn't mean it's safer to eat raw oysters, as most of us know.

The American Society for Microbiology (ASM) warns of numerous dangers in eating seafood, while stressing the benefits derived from seafood consumption. "Contamination of seafood by pathogens with a human reservoir can occur when growing areas are contaminated with human sewage. Outbreaks of seafood-associated illness linked to polluted waters have been caused by calicivirus, hepatitis A virus, and Salmonella Enterica serotype Typhi," according to the ASM.[12]

> Identified sources of seafood contamination have included overboard sewage discharged into harvest areas, illegal harvesting from sewage-contaminated waters, and sewage runoff from points inland after heavy rains or flooding. Additionally, seafood may become contaminated during handling, processing, or preparation. Contributing factors may include storage and transportation at inappropriate temperatures, contamination by an infected food handler, or cross-contamination through contact with contaminated seafood or seawater. Adequate cooking kills most pathogens; however, unlike other foods, such as meat and poultry, that are usually fully cooked, seafood is often consumed raw or prepared in ways that do not kill organisms.[13]

We do not know how extensive seafood poisonings stretch, the exact number of illnesses involved, or how many cases go unreported. The ASM's *Clinical Microbiology Review* explains this difficult problem: "Our analysis of surveillance data is subject to several limitations. The true burden of illnesses associated with seafood consumption is probably much greater than what we report. Our understanding of foods and pathogens responsible for illness is largely derived from information gained from outbreak investigations."[14]

However, many outbreaks likely go unrecognized and uninvestigated. Moreover, the Foodborne Disease Outbreak Online Database Surveillance System, a passive agency developed by the CDC, relies on voluntary reporting, which may lead to further underestimation of the actual number of outbreaks and illnesses that occur.[15] Outbreak reporting may not be uniform across states, which may be due in part to whether states have dedicated foodborne disease epidemiologists. Also, outbreaks comprise only a small proportion of all cases of foodborne illness.

It's not unlikely that eating raw oysters and raw fish, particularly uncooked salmon, can cause serious illness and even death. Many people still eat raw oysters, ignoring the risk of contracting foodborne illnesses such as Vibrio parahaemolyticus.[16] And most of them have no intention of removing raw oysters from their diet.

Fish Frauds

The FDA continues to find certain Chinese seafood imported to the United States to contain illegal substances. The problem originates in the fish farming industry. Check the labels for "farm raised" as opposed to the preferred "wild caught," a much safer way to eat fish and shellfish. Much of the seafood from China reaches us contaminated with antimicrobial agents that are banned in the United States. Nitrofurans, malachite green, and gentian violet have been shown to cause cancer with long-term exposure in lab animals. Keep in mind much of this contaminated seafood continues to reach dinner tables due to the lack of inspections of imported foods by the FDA.

A California importer recalled more than 58,000 pounds of tuna scrape in early 2012 after the product was linked to an outbreak of Salmonella bareilly that sickened at least 425 people in 28 states. The outbreak sent 55 people to hospitals. No deaths were reported. Tuna scrape is meat scraped from the bones of the fish and was included in the production of spicy tuna sushi rolls that "likely" caused the illnesses. At the time, public health officials alerted retailers that because the raw tuna was separated into smaller lots, some of it might still be in freezers. The raw tuna scrape linked to the illnesses was traced to imports from India.

Oceana, founded in 2001, calls itself the largest international organization focused solely on ocean conservation. In 2013 the organization set about a project to determine the extent of illegal labeling of fish and other frauds connected to seafood.[17] In the investigation, Oceana took 1,200 samples of seafood between 2010 and 2012 from U.S. restaurants and stores. DNA testing was performed at the University of Guelph's Canadian Centre for DNA. The findings show that

- Thirty-three percent of the samples were mislabeled.
- Fish was wrongly marketed as snapper in 87 percent of cases.
- Tuna was fraudulent 59 percent of the time.
- Halibut, grouper, cod, and Chilean sea bass proved fake 19 percent to 38 percent of the time.
- Expensive fish such as tilapia was replaced with farmed red snapper.

The National Oceanic and Atmospheric Administration (NOAA) investigates fish fraud under the Lacey Act, which makes the traffic of illegally gained fish a federal crime.

One problem in tracing the fraud is exacerbated by the overwhelming majority of imported fish not carrying a Country of Origin Label (COOL). The label is not required on minimally processed seafood.

Catfish

Let's talk about catfish, those lowly bottom feeders, and our love-hate relationship with this mud cat. Depending on the part of country you live in or visit you might hear them called "polliwogs" or "chuckleheads." Scientifically, they are Siluriformes from the Animalia kingdom.

Catfish raising constitutes a major part of the U.S. fish industry, especially in the South. However, catfish imports increase every year, jumping from 2 percent of the U.S. market to 23 percent of the market in the eight-year period ending in 2010. The 2008 farm bill moved the responsibility of enforcement and inspections from the FDA to the USDA, giving catfish producers in the United States an advantage over foreign producers, who will now have to conform to the same standards as U.S. catfish-raisers. The problem with this strategy is that there have been no more complaints or illnesses from imported catfish than from those produced in the United States.

You knew sooner or later we would have to get around to the politics of seafood in the United States. But you didn't suspect the subject would be the whiskered catfish. The folks over at Politico.com published an opinion piece from Senator John McCain (R-AZ) in June 2013.[18] "What makes catfish so special? It turns out that catfish farmers in Mississippi, Alabama and Arkansas are having a difficult time selling their crusty mudcats to consumers," McCain said.

When American families dine on shrimp, tilapia, or the occasional fried catfish, they tend to prefer good-tasting seafood at the best prices, which general-

ly comes from the vast supply of imported Asian seafood. Rather than compete, southern catfish farmers asked their powerful friends, the senators from
Michigan and Mississippi, to support a law in the Farm Bill that forces
Americans to buy domestic catfish. They want you to think Americans have
been eating unsafe foreign catfish (it's just catfish, of course) even though the
FDA, the CDC, and the USDA itself say that's untrue. Out of the 1.8 billion
catfish enjoyed by Americans each year, only two illnesses are reported on
average.

McCain added a final note: "This is one fishy deal that needs to be fried on
behalf of the American taxpayer."

The General Accountability Office (GAO) disagrees with moving the
inspection duties, saying it will cost taxpayers more and add to the already
fragmented food safety bureaucracy. Will the move cut down on foodborne
illnesses? More inspections are mandated for the imported catfish, but the
United States is already dangerously short of inspectors and every year
checks fewer and fewer of the imports.

A few weeks after Senator McCain's opinion piece was published, the
Senate approved a farm bill that did not include the suggestions from
McCain and the GAO.

Safe to Eat

I'm sure by now you're wondering if there is any fish in the seven seas and
all the oceans, rivers, and streams that is safe to eat. Health officials advise us
to select fish and shellfish known to have low levels of mercury: wild Alaska
and Pacific salmon, striped bass, sturgeon, Pacific flounder, anchovies, herring, crawfish, king crab, and scallops.[19] And if you're on the lookout for fish
high in Omega-3 fatty acids, try sardines, with 1,950 mg per three-ounce
serving. They're also high in protein and vitamin D, plus they're low in
mercury and toxins.

I checked with our friends over at the Organic Consumers Association in
Finland, Minnesota.[20] They categorize the safer seafood according to the
level of mercury:

- *Low mercury*: anchovies, Arctic char, Pacific flounder, herring, king crab,
  sand dabs (abundant on the Pacific coast), scallops, Pacific sole, tilapia,
  wild Alaska and Pacific salmon, farmed catfish, clams, striped bass, and
  sturgeon
- *Moderate mercury*: Alaskan halibut, black cod, blue (Gulf Coast) crab,
  cod, Dungeness crab, Eastern oysters, mahi-mahi, blue mussels, Pollack,
  and tuna (canned light)

When it comes to young children, pregnant women, nursing mothers, and women of childbearing age, they refer to the FDA and EPA guidelines: Eat no more than two or three meals, or 12 ounces total, of fish or shellfish a week, and limit high-mercury fish to one serving per week. Those of you in this category should avoid escolar, mackerel, marlin, and orange roughy.

Salmon, especially Coho and Alaskan, makes most lists of safe and healthy seafood. Also, wild-caught Dungeness crab, sardines, and squid are recommended.[21]

Every year since 1993, the EPA has made available to the public a compendium of information on locally issued fish advisories, consumption advisories, and safe eating guidelines.[22] They have you covered just about anywhere you live or travel, all states, U.S. territories, and even Indian reservations. Don't forget to check with local governments as well (e.g., your state's Parks and Wildlife Department).

Chapter Nine

Deli Dangers

If you must shop for your meat and cheese at a delicatessen, please make your selections from the prepackaged items. If you choose to have the meat sliced at the deli, you risk eating food that has a higher likelihood of containing Listeria—nearly five times higher than prepackaged meats of the same quality.[1] The CDC stated, "Between 2009–2011, the agency logged in 1,650 illnesses from Listeria monocytogenes along with 1,500 hospitalizations, and 260 deaths. Compared with other major foodborne diseases, Listeriosis' fatality rate ranks very high, hospitalization extremely high, but the disease is relatively rare."[2]

Deli meat ranks as containing the third-highest combination of food and disease-causing microorganisms, according to the University of Florida's Emerging Pathogens Institute.[3] A USDA public meeting in 2009 concluded that 83 percent of the illnesses and deaths from Listeria monocytogenes in deli food consumption are attributed to deli meat sliced and packaged at the retail level, that is, the meat counter at your grocery store or the neighborhood deli.[4]

In the United States, Listeriosis, one of the most deadly diseases, carries a fatality rate of 21 percent, compared with only 0.5 percent for Salmonella or E. coli O157:H7. Perhaps the serious dangers of Listeriosis can be better described this way: One in every five persons infected with Listeria dies.

Why are delis so dangerous? High-risk foods such as deli meats, soft cheeses, pate, and smoked seafood account for 67 percent of food contaminations. Here's why: Throughout the day, the meats and cheeses are pushed through slicers that often are not cleaned until the end of the day. And a slicer designated for meat only may have been used for cheese or another meat that has cross-contaminated the slicer, allowing the quick spread of any pathogens to meats purchased by other customers.[5]

Cross-contamination of Listeria monocytogenes in the retail environment dramatically increases the predicted risk of Listeriosis and is not amenable to a simple solution, according to the FDA.[6] In other words, attempts to solve the problem leave inspectors at a loss. The lack of proper hand washing presents another real danger to retail-sliced meats and cheeses. FDA investigators also noted inadequate temperatures of refrigeration units and meats left on cutting boards too long during busy periods of the day.

A 2013 study by the USDA consisted of 50 visits to delis by investigators who checked food temperatures, possible cross-contamination on meat and cheese slicers, and personal hygiene of employees. The investigators noted that 60 percent of the delis visited failed to hold food at 41 degrees or below as required by the FDA Food Code. In all 50 of the delis checked, at least one employee failed to wash their hands as required, even when the inspectors were visibly present.[7]

Federal guidelines simply state, "Wearing gloves while serving customers reduces the estimated risk of Listeriosis." But the FDA failed to mention the obvious: If the gloves become contaminated from handling one product, and the employee then moves to another product without changing gloves, the second product potentially becomes contaminated along with other products handled with the same gloves.

Jennifer C. McEntire, PhD, vice president and chief science officer at the Acheson Group, agrees. "Contaminated gloves transfer pathogens, as do contaminated slicers, niches are bad, sanitation is important and temperature is important."[8] McEntire spent eight years as a senior staff scientist at the Institute of Food Technologists (IFT). She realizes deli food may have become contaminated prior to reaching the retailer.[9] "The coolest, cleanest deli cannot counter the risk associated with a product that has been contaminated at the level of the manufacturer. Nor can the greatest controls in manufacturing negate poor sanitation and handling practices at the retail food service level," she says.

Michael Batz, writing in the *Wall Street Journal*'s health blog, says many of the conditions found behind the deli counter are conducive to Listeria, which, unlike other organisms, can grow in the refrigerator.[10] "It can be spread by worker's hands and colonize in cracks, food preparation areas and food-filled crevices on meat and cheese slicers, which is a challenge to sanitation procedures." He advises consumers to keep their own refrigerators extremely clean and to eat deli meats within three or four days, or by the date stamped on the package at the point of purchase. "From the minute you buy deli meats, there's a window of opportunity for things to get in there," says Batz.

The USDA advises that cleaning and sanitizing food contact surfaces reduces the predicted Listeria levels in the deli area. One of the first things certified food sanitarians learned in their training is something called "time and temperature." How long has the potentially hazardous food been left on the cutting block and at what temperature? If perishable food has been above 41 degrees for more than two hours, throw it out. If you're uncertain about the length of time, discard the food anyway. The clock is ticking and the temperature is rising as clerks busily wait on other customers, while the Listeria bacteria waits for no one.

One way to avoid the dangers in the deli is to stay away, for many reasons. Seriously! When nitrates and sodium from deli meats mix together in the stomach they can turn into a carcinogenic compound traced to cancers. Eating processed foods like cold cuts can raise your risk for colorectal cancer. Any meat, sausage, hot dogs, roast beef, pepperoni, and beef jerky becomes "processed" once it has been preserved.[11] Sodium nitrate added to many processed meats enhances the appearance of the meats and makes them last longer. The USDA tried to ban sodium nitrates from processed meats back in the 1970s. The big meat industry and its paid lobbyists fought the proposed ban and won.[12] It's just another example of our government playing into the hands of big business and snubbing the critical needs of consumers.

"Research shows that eating processed meats, like bacon and cold cuts, can raise your risk for colorectal cancer," says Mary Ellen Herndon, a wellness dietitian at the University of Texas MD Anderson Cancer Center.[13] "That's because cancer-causing substances form when meats are preserved. And, eating these substances can damage your DNA," she added in a July 2013 article on the MD Anderson website. In addition to bacon and cold cuts and the aforementioned meats, other processed foods include sausage and wieners.

Eating deli turkey meat caused an outbreak of Listeria monocytogenes in 10 states in 2000, sickening 29 people, and was associated with four deaths and three miscarriages/stillbirths.[14]

In May 2011 the American Institute for Cancer released a study that also ties processed meats to an increase in the risk of developing colorectal cancer.[15] A person who eats 3.5 ounces of processed meat every day has a 36 percent higher risk of developing cancer than a person who eats no processed meat.

Women's Health magazine says a daily dose of 50 grams, about two slices of processed red meats such as bologna and salami, increases heart disease risk by 42 percent and diabetes risk by 19 percent.[16] High amounts of nitrates (and sodium) may explain the higher risk of heart attacks and diabetes. Pregnant women are about 20 percent more likely than other healthy adults to get Listeriosis; newborns suffer the most serious effects of infection in pregnancy, according to the CDC.[17] If you are pregnant, the CDC clearly states, "Do not eat hot dogs, luncheon meats, cold cuts or other deli meats unless they are heated to an internal temperature of 165°F or until steaming hot. Do not eat these foods from a deli or meat counter: refrigerated pate, meat spreads, soft cheese such as feta, queso blanco, queso fresco, brie, camembert or blue veined cheese. Do not eat refrigerated smoked seafood, unless it is contained in a cooked dish, such as a casserole, or unless it is a canned or a shelf stable product. Refrigerated smoked seafood, such as salmon, trout, whitefish, cod, tuna, and mackerel, is most often labeled as 'nova style,' 'lox,' 'kippered,' 'smoked,' or 'jerky' and must not be eaten if you are pregnant. Canned and shelf stable tuna, salmon, and other fish products are safe to eat."

The World Cancer Research Fund (WCRF) advises consumers "to reduce your cancer risk, eat no more than 500 g (cooked weight) per week of red meat, like beef, pork and lamb, and avoid processed meats such as ham, bacon, salami, hot dogs and some sausages."[18]

A Biomedcentral (BMC) Medicine study estimated that "3.3% (95% CI 1.5% to 5.0%) of deaths could be prevented if all participants had a processed meat consumption of less than 20 grams a day. Significant associations with processed meat intake were observed for cardiovascular diseases, cancer, and other causes of death."[19]

Consumers should be aware of Listeria in dairy products, including queso fresco, which often is made with unpasteurized milk. Pregnant women are about 10 times more likely than other healthy adults to become ill from Listeriosis. Fetuses, not the mother, suffer the most during pregnancy with Listeriosis.

When Listeria contamination is discovered, recalls of the product usually take place within hours or a few days. In the spring of 2013, Manda Packing Company recalled almost 500 pounds of ham shanks, turkey breast, roast beef, tasso pork, hog head cheese, pastrami, and corned beef, according to the USDA.[20] The meats, recalled due to possible contamination with Listeria monocytogenes, had been shipped to delis and other retail stores across 13 states.

The CDC stated that between 2009 and 2011, the agency logged 1,650 illnesses from Listeria monocytogenes, along with 1,500 hospitalizations and 260 deaths. Compared with other major foodborne diseases, the fatality rate of Listeriosis ranks very high and hospitalization from illness extremely high, although the disease is relatively rare. Of the 10 outbreaks with an identified food source, six were linked to soft cheese (mostly Mexican-style cheeses) according to the CDC.

It would seem inconceivable that two U.S. Food Safety agencies, the USDA and the FDA, could have two contrasting rules regarding the presence of Listeria in foods. Chris Waldrop, director of the Food Policy Institute of the Consumer Federation of America (CFA) (and an extremely determined and patient man) pointed out a major discrepancy between the USDA and the FDA. He tried getting his point across to the two leading food safety arms of our government in an April 2008 letter.[21] Nothing happened. He also mentioned the subject in June 2013 without any results.

Here's the problem: The U.S. Food Safety and Inspection Service of the USDA conducted a comparative risk assessment study for Listeria monocytogenes in ready-to-eat meat packaged at food processing plants and retail deli sliced meat. It stated that "for ready-to-eat (RTE) foods that do not support the growth of Listeria, FDA would regard the food as adulterated when Listeria is present at or above 100 cfu/g of food. This is in contrast to the USDA's policy, which maintains a zero tolerance for Listeria in RTE foods."

Waldrop points to insufficient labeling of retail ready-to-eat foods. "The federal government, in its food safety education materials, advises pregnant women to thoroughly reheat certain RTE foods such as hot dogs and deli meats. It also advises pregnant women to avoid soft cheeses, pate, smoked fish, and unpasteurized milk," Waldrop said.

Labels on ready-to-eat deli foods "could include the same language used in the federal government's food safety education materials, such as: 'If you are pregnant or immune suppressed, reheat this product to steaming hot or 165°F before eating.' Placing this message on the package would assure that the information was immediately available at the time of purchase as well as consumption, and would help remind susceptible individuals that the product is not 'ready-to-eat' and should be handled appropriately," he added.

The CFA in December 2004 published a scathing report called "Not Ready to Eat," describing how the meat and poultry industry allegedly weakened efforts to reduce Listeria food poisoning.[22] According to a portion of the CFA's executive summary of the report:

> During the Bush Administration's first term, the approach taken by the USDA to controlling Listeria shifted significantly to favor positions taken by the regulated industry. The Department first delayed regulations to control Listeria contamination in ready-to-eat meat and poultry products and then revised them to reflect industry positions. During the same period, the government abandoned its pledge to reduce by 50 percent the number of Listeria food-poisoning (Listeriosis) cases by 2005. These events raise the question of whether a 22 percent increase in Listeria food-poisoning cases in 2003 can be attributed, at least in part, to the change in USDA policy and approach.[23]

The CFA also stated, "While reading a report filled with numbers and charts, it is easy to get mired in the statistics and technical terminology of food-safety regulation and the speeches of self-serving industry and public officials who can find a way to spin a success story from the most dismal performance."[24] But it is critical to remember that the statistics of deaths and illnesses represent real people—some of them very young—who are the real losers here.

One of those was tiny Matthew Wysocki, born several weeks premature by emergency cesarean due to Listeria food poisoning.[25] He laid in intensive care for six days, attached to every imaginable piece of neonatal lifesaving equipment. When the infection began attacking his brain, his parents decided to remove him from life support. His father held his tiny body, and Matthew opened his eyes and struggled to breathe on his own. Then he died.

Why did Matthew have to suffer this way? Because the meat and poultry industry and USDA too often forget their responsibility to the people they serve, and because Matthew's pregnant mother ate "ready-to-eat" cold cuts that were neither ready nor safe to eat.

Chapter Ten

Outbreaks, Illnesses, and Deaths

Scores of known pathogens can cause you to become sick from eating contaminated food. Salmonella, the leading cause of illnesses from known pathogens, represents only one of the more than 200 diseases transmitted through food.[1] Some foods simply carry more foodborne diseases than others. Many magazines annually publish their idea of the most dangerous foods, based on government data on foodborne illnesses and other sources. *Men's Health* magazine lists chicken, ground beef, ground turkey, raw oysters, cantaloupe, peaches, prepackaged lettuce, cold cuts (deli meat), scallions, and eggs, in that order, as most susceptible to pathogens.[2]

(The numbers of illnesses from foodborne pathogens are only estimates. For example, sporadic illnesses caused by the pathogens Bacillus cereus, Clostridium perfringens, and Staphylococcus aureus are not reported. These cases are counted only during outbreaks. CDC assumed that if diagnosed sporadic cases were reported, the total number would be 10 ten times the number of outbreak-related cases.[3] Many of the foodborne illnesses are not reported because the ill person does not seek medical care, the health-care provider does not obtain a specimen for diagnosis, the laboratory does not perform the necessary diagnostic test, or the illnesses or laboratory findings are not communicated to public health officials. To obtain an estimate, CDC calculates the difference between the number of reported cases and the number of cases that actually occur in the community. For Salmonella, the under-reporting has been estimated at about 38-fold, for E. coli O157:H7 about 20, and for Campylobacter about 38; for Listeria monocytogenes, CDC "arbitrarily used a far lower multiplier of 2, on the assumption that most cases come to medical attention." The numbers of hospitalizations and deaths, obviously, are much more precise.)

The U.S. Centers for Disease Control and Prevention compiled a list of the six most deadly foodborne pathogens, based on a decade long study from 1998 to 2008. Heading the list is Salmonella.[4] Second is Listeria, followed by E. coli O157:H7, Hepatitis A, Clostridium Perfringens, and Rotavius. These pathogens are extremely critical and must be included when discussing foodborne illnesses, hospitalizations, and death. We'll discuss each one of these disease-causing agents with some examples of documented cases.

THE SIX DEADLIEST FOODBORNE PATHOGENS

Salmonella

About 1.2 million people become ill every year from Salmonella. Nearly 23,000 are hospitalized, and 450 die. The illness caused by the bacteria is Salmonellosis. Symptoms include diarrhea, fever, and abdominal cramps beginning about 12 to 72 hours after infection. The CDC says most people recover without treatment, but in some the diarrhea may be so severe that the patient needs to be hospitalized. Children are the most likely to get Salmonellosis.

Chrissy Christoferson appeared before the USDA on July 25, 2013, and related how her 10-month-old son, Beck, became a statistic with the FDA and CDC. It was easy. He only had to eat a Veggie Booty, a snack his mother thought was a healthy choice.[5] But the snack contained a spice that may have been the source of Salmonella wandsworth, which sickened 65 people in 20 states in 2007.

When Beck showed signs of the flu, Chrissy noticed layers of skin falling off his body during diaper changes, She took him to their pediatrician for an exam. His stool contained blood and mucus. During Beck's 10-day illness, doctors confirmed the source of the infection. Chrissy wondered what struggles her son could experience in later life. His body was still developing; the health impacts were unknown. Six years passed and Chrissy still didn't know the full impact of this foodborne disease.[6]

What you have just read is just part of the story Chrissy told the FDA on July 25, 2013. Chrissy emphasized the need for full implementation of the proposed Food Safety Modernization Act, or FSMA. The act would help prevent outbreaks like this one from occurring and help ensure that food processors ship only safe food by implementing various preventative controls, including testing.

Monika Samaan, a seven-year-old Australian girl, sickened by Salmonella poisoning from a chicken wrap at Kentucky Fried Chicken in 2005, remained in a coma for months with severe brain damage.[7] New South Wales Supreme Court Justice Stephen Rothman ordered KFC to pay AU $8 million in damages plus legal costs.[8]

It's difficult to imagine almost a quarter of a million people getting sick on ice cream.[9] But in September 1994, failure to clean a transport tanker of nonpasteurized liquid eggs containing Salmonella enteritidis led to the contamination of its next shipment of clean premix.[10] More than 224,000 were sickened after eating Schwan's ice cream containing the Salmonella enteritidis. The Minnesota Department of Health said shipping pasteurized products in dedicated containers could prevent similar outbreaks in the future.

Tainted post-pasteurized milk from Hillfarm Dairy in Melrose Park, Illinois, caused 16,284 confirmed cases of food poisoning in 1985.[11] Add the unreported cases and the number probably totaled 200,000 cases, according to the CDC.[12] Salmonella typhimurium was responsible for two deaths and may have been related to the death of four or five others with some counts being as high as 12. At the time, it was considered the largest outbreak of Salmonella food poisoning recorded in U.S. history.[13]

In 1989, Salmonella chester sickened approximately 25,000 people in 30 states in the United States after eating cantaloupes imported from Mexico.[14] Also, in 2011, Salmonella enteritis sickened 68 people who ate at Mexican-style quick-service restaurants across 10 states.[15] The public outcry shifted from the food poisoning to the steadfast refusal by the CDC to name the restaurant chain involved in the illnesses. The feds called it "a chain of Mexican restaurants." Beyond that you had to guess where to eat and where not to eat, which is unfair to all the chains not involved. The CDC continued for months its refusal to identify the restaurant chain despite the widespread illnesses. People complained that they could not eat at any fast food Mexican restaurant, not knowing which one was the culprit under investigation.

Finally, weeks later, after a lot of digging by scores of reporters, a document was found at the Oklahoma State Department of Health's Acute Disease Service.[16] That document named Taco Bell as the chain at which the contamination was found. Taco Bell officials stated that they had been assured by the CDC that public health was not at risk and the incident was completely over. The CDC continued its silence on naming the chain.

The year prior to this outbreak, Taco Bell was linked to a Salmonella outbreak that sickened 155 people in 21 states.[17] And in 2006, contaminated lettuce served at Taco Bell restaurants in the northeast United States caused an E. coli outbreak that sickened more than 70 people.[18] No deaths were reported.

So why did the CDC fail to immediately name Taco Bell as the chain involved in the outbreak? CDC's policy, in part, is: "If there's not an important public health reason to use the name publicly, CDC doesn't use the name publicly."[19] That policy goes along with the longstanding belief by many that the CDC, FDA, and USDA many times try harder to protect businesses than to protect the health of the public.

Listeria Monocytogenes

Listeriosis is second in the CDC listing of deadliest foodborne illnesses. Almost all Listeriosis occurs in persons in higher-risk groups, according to the CDC. The most prominent vehicle carrying the pathogen is soft cheeses. Listeriosis usually is a mild illness in pregnant women, but it can cause severe outcomes for the fetus or newborn infant. [20]

The FDA and Health Canada estimate that the risk for Listeriosis from soft-ripened cheeses is 50 to 160 times higher per serving when the cheese has been made with unpasteurized (raw) milk rather than pasteurized milk. [21]

The deadliest Listeria outbreak in the United States resulted in 52 recorded deaths in southern California in 1985. [22] The victims ate Listeria-contaminated Mexican-style cheeses made by Jalisco in California. Considering the number of deaths, the outbreak became the deadliest foodborne illness event in the United States since the 1970s, when tracking began. The deaths included 19 stillbirths, 10 infant deaths, and 20 miscarriages.

The bacterial disease Listeriosis causes meningitis and sepsis, especially in persons with an impaired immune system. Pregnant women may also transmit the infection to their infants, resulting in abortion or early neonatal sepsis. People living in southern California's large Mexican American community sustained the largest percentage of deaths and illnesses.

The CDC found that Jalisco used a nonlicensed technician to pasteurize the milk and may have diluted the product with raw (nonpasteurized) milk. [23] The cheese caused 142 cases of Listeriosis.

Listeria caused the illnesses of more than 3,500 people during outbreaks from 2010 through 2012. Recalls during the outbreaks involved 550 million eggs from two Iowa farms and another million eggs in 34 states. [24] Sara Lee Corporation's subsidiary, Bil Mar Foods, was named as the source of the Listeria monocytogenes that killed at least 21 people and sickened 100 others. [25] Sara Lee recalled 35 million pounds of hot dogs and deli meats. The Sara Lee plant in Zeeland, Michigan, had been tested in July 1998 after the facility replaced a refrigeration unit. Condensation appeared. During the next few weeks, 11 out of 12 samples proved positive for bacteria. The plant tried to clean up. The USDA sent out four dozen noncompliance warnings threatening administrative actions, but the USDA took no action until it was too late. Tests for pathogens made by the company continued to come back high. The company stopped testing in November 1998, a month before the Sara Lee recall.

Peter Perl of the *Washington Post* asked, "Why didn't the U.S. Department of Agriculture blow the whistle sooner on Sara Lee?" [26] Perl had good reason to ask the question. Bil Mar accumulated 287 citations for federal food safety violations.

The potentially deadly Listeria monocytogenes began taking its toll. Within two months, 21 people had died from eating Sara Lee BallPark franks. The USDA had not acted and even failed to issue a news release, as its policies require, notifying the public of the danger. Instead, as the *Washington Post* pointed out, "the USDA relied on an announcement issued by Bil Mar that did not mention the full scope of the recall or the dire nature of the illness, let alone the deaths."

Once again we see our government deciding to protect big business rather than following the law and placing the protection of consumers first.

In 1985, Listeria tainted Mexican cheese made by a Los Angeles company killed 28 people and sickened scores of others, mostly women, many who were pregnant. And in 2002, sliced turkey meats from Pilgrim's Pride killed eight people. While probing the cause of an outbreak that forced the recall of 27 million pounds of turkey and chicken products, investigators from the USDA found extensive amounts of Listeria in all parts of Pilgrim's Pride's Wampler Foods plant in Franconia, Pennsylvania.[27] Seven people died, 46 were sickened, and three miscarriages occurred from eating the turkey deli meat. Pilgrim's Pride, based in Pittsburg, Texas, is the country's second-largest poultry producer.

It's important to point out again that Listeria monocytogenes, a serious and sometimes fatal infection, can cause miscarriages and stillbirths among pregnant women, according to the FDA. The disease primarily affects older adults, pregnant women, newborns, and adults with weakened immune systems.

More than 30 people died and over 100 sickened, many of them hospitalized, in a foodborne spread of illness in 2011 that food safety experts say could have been prevented. Listeria-contaminated Rocky Ford cantaloupes were grown at the 6,000-acre Jensen Farms in Eastern Colorado near the town of Holly.[28] Brothers Ryan and Eric Jensen inherited the farm that had been handed down through three previous generations. They made some changes to the operation, including the removal of the antimicrobial wash. As CNN's investigative reporters discovered, "Without the antimicrobial wash, melons that pass along the packing equipment are placed in pools of water to rinse and cross-contaminate one another, and an entire production line can spread dangerous bacteria."[29]

An FDA report stated that "several areas on both the washing and drying equipment appeared to be un-cleanable" and an old washing machine redesigned for cleaning potatoes had been substituted to clean the melons.[30]

No federal food safety agency inspects cantaloupes. Like so many other foods—fish, produce, meat, and other food products—too few inspectors and too many food sources means that few food products receive testing or inspection. The CNN investigation concluded: "Most troubling of all, virtually nothing is in place, no protective systems that could prevent this from happening again, someplace else."

E. coli O157:H7

This third most deadly foodborne pathogen caused 22 deaths in the 308 outbreaks included in the study. E. coli O157:H7 bacteria can cause severe abdominal cramps, bloody diarrhea, and vomiting. The infection may originate in contaminated water or food, particularly in undercooked ground beef and raw vegetables. Young children and older adults can develop hemolytic uremic syndrome (HUS), which is a life-threatening form of kidney failure. Healthy adults usually recover within a week.[31]

The CDC provides a detailed description of how E. coli infections spread. This may help you avoid the pathogen by simply knowing and applying the following information.

Infections start when you swallow tiny, usually invisible amounts of human or animal feces in your mouth. "This happens more often than we would like to think about," says the CDC. "Exposures that result in illness include consumption of contaminated food, consumption of unpasteurized (raw) milk, consumption of water that has not been disinfected, contact with cattle, or contact with the feces of infected people."

The contact is pretty obvious like changing a diaper, cows at a dairy, but sometimes it is not so apparent. "People have gotten infected by swallowing lake water while swimming, touching the environment in petting zoos and other animal exhibits, and by eating food prepared by people who did not wash their hands well after using the toilet. Almost everyone has some risk of infection," according to the CDC.

This country saw its first deadly foodborne E. coli O157:H7 outbreak in 1993 when four children died and 700 others were infected after eating undercooked hamburgers at a Jack in the Box restaurant. In recent years, E. coli has been linked to U.S. outbreaks involving sprouts, lettuce, hazelnuts, beef, prepackaged cookie dough, spinach, and pizza.[32]

Hepatitis A

Much like E. coli O157:H7, foodborne Hepatitis A can be transmitted by the fecal-oral route either by direct contact with a carrier of Hepatitis A virus or by ingestion of the virus contaminated food or water, according to the CDC.[33] The median time from exposure to onset of symptoms is 28 days. "Hepatitis A begins with symptoms such as fever, anorexia, nausea, vomiting, diarrhea, myalgia, and malaise. Jaundice dark-colored urine, or light-colored stools might be present at onset or might follow constitutional symptoms within a few days," according to the CDC. Hepatitis A lasts for several weeks.

In 2003, the largest foodborne hepatitis outbreak in U.S. history killed three and infected 555 who ate contaminated green onions at a Chi Chi's restaurant in Monaca, Pennsylvania.[34]

At least 13 Chi Chi's food service workers and 75 residents of six other states who dined at the restaurant were sickened. Immune globulin was provided to about 9,000 persons who ate from the restaurant between September 14 and October 17, 2003.

The green onions were grown, harvested, and processed in northern Mexico near the U.S. border, according to the FDA.[35]

During the 10-year period of the CDC study, eight deaths from Hepatitis A were reported within 76 outbreaks.

Clostridium Perfringens

Clostridium perfringens, little known to the average person, often resides on raw meat and poultry. The bacterium is found in many environmental sources as well as in the intestines of humans and animals. Conditions with little or no oxygen stimulate growth and under ideal conditions can multiply rapidly. C. Perfringens is one of the most common causes of foodborne illnesses in the United States, according to the CDC. The agency logs in nearly a million cases of foodborne sicknesses each year from C. Perfringens.

The pathogen struck 42 residents and 12 staff members at a Louisiana State Psychiatric Hospital in May 2010.[36] Three of the patients died within 24 hours. The Louisiana Office of Public Health found that eating chicken served at dinner the night before was associated with the illness. The chicken was cooked about 24 hours before serving and not cooled in accordance with hospital guidelines.

A 46-year-old woman was one of 30 diners to fall ill after eating a four-course Christmas Day lunch at the Railway Hotel in Hornchurch, Essex, in January 2013.

After being taken to a hospital, Della Callagher was sent home and told to lie down. Others affected by the illness improved, but Ms. Callagher's condition grew worse. Her husband called an ambulance, she was admitted to a hospital, and died the next day. The Health Protection Agency later confirmed that she had contracted Clostridium Perfringens that strikes about 90,000 Britons a year.[37]

In the CDC survey from 1998 to 2008, lists this pathogen as the fourth deadliest in the nation. Eight people died in the 536 outbreaks during that decade.[38]

Rotavirus

People who get rotavirus disease can become severely dehydrated, need to be hospitalized, and can even die.[39] The virus can cause inflammation of the stomach and intestines, severe watery diarrhea, often with vomiting, fever, and abdominal pain. There is no antiviral drug to treat rotavirus infection. Antibiotic drugs will not help because antibiotics fight against bacteria not viruses.[40]

Prior to the introduction of a rotavirus vaccine in 2006, rotavirus was the leading cause of severe diarrhea among infants and young children in the United States. Up until that time, almost all children in this country were infected with rotavirus before the age of five. This resulted in 55,000 to 70,000 hospitalizations and 20 to 60 deaths each year.

The disease in the United States peaked in the winter and spring months, usually beginning in the Southwest part of the country and moving Northeast. The pattern is no longer consistent since the vaccine became available in 2006.[41]

"Millions of United States infants have received the rotavirus vaccine since it became available in 2006. Rotavirus disease among infants and young children has since decreased significantly in the United States," the CDC reports.[42]

Globally, rotavirus remains a major medical problem. In 2008, rotavirus caused an estimated 453,000 deaths worldwide in children younger than five years of age, according to the CDC.[43]

Seven deaths were reported to the CDC in ten outbreaks of Rotavirus poisonings during the 10-year survey period.

Norovirus

A pathogen that failed to reach the top six made headlines because of its popularity. "Norovirus is so common, the Health District doesn't bother keeping stats on it," reads a headline in *Las Vegas, Nevada City Life* in 2013.[44] Norovirus cases strike 20 million people every year in the United States, killing 800 and hospitalizing another 70,000, according to the CDC.[45] Cruise ships frequently report major outbreaks of the highly contagious Norovirus, with hundreds of people becoming ill within a few hours. Foodborne outbreaks in hospitals almost always turn up Norovirus as the cause. The incidents of Norovirus cases increased dramatically from 1995 to the present. Here are some of the incidents of sicknesses, mostly Norovirus, reported to the CDC.[46]

- The Royal Caribbean Cruise Line's Explorer of the Seas in January 2014, experienced the worst outbreak of Norovirus on a cruise ship when 626 passengers and 50 crew members became ill.[47]
- Celebrity Cruises reported 443 sickened from Norovirus in February 2010.
- Another Celebrity Cruises ship a month later experienced a Norovirus outbreak that sickened 419.
- Princess Cruises' Crown Princess reported in January 2010 that 396 passengers became ill from Norovirus.
- Two years later, 363 passengers and crew members contracted Norovirus aboard the Crown Princess.
- The Fred Olsen Cruise Lines was hit with a Norovirus outbreak 15 days before ending its world cruise. The sicknesses affected 293 passengers and 17 crew members.
- The Ruby Princess Eastern Caribbean cruise to Fort Lauderdale, Florida, experienced 271 sicknesses from the Norovirus pathogen.
- In February 2009 the Coral Princess had the distinction of sickening passengers with E. coli as well as Norovirus.
- Norovirus struck 265 people on board the Carnival Liberty in April 2009.
- The Voyager of the Seas was delayed at various ports for sanitization after 259 passengers and crew members were sickened with Norovirus.
- The Cunard Line Queen Mary 2 was hit with 220 cases of Norovirus during its December 2012 cruise.
- The Sun Princess experienced 216 Norovirus illnesses during a cruise in July 2012.

Symptoms of Norovirus include diarrhea, vomiting, nausea, stomach pain, fever, and headache. The CDC refers to the pathogen as the ubiquitous Norovirus. It's among the most infectious virus known to man and can be transmitted through inanimate objects such as reusable grocery bags.[48] Made from woven polypropylene, the popular bags replace the plastic bags that clog our streams and landfills. The first-ever case of transmitting Norovirus through a reusable grocery bag sickened seven young soccer players in Oregon. The first girl stricken had gone to a restroom and placed a grocery bag of cookies on the floor near the door. The girl vomited in a toilet and the virus spread through the air about 10 feet, contaminating the bag of cookies. The other players became ill after eating the cookies.

Toxoplasmosis, a Parasite

Turning now to the parasite of most concern to the CDC, Toxoplasmosis. It's one of the leading causes of death attributed to foodborne illness in the United States. Women newly infected with Toxoplasma during pregnancy and anyone with a compromised immune system should be aware that Toxoplasmosis can have severe consequences. [49]

One of the greatest dangers of contracting Toxoplasmosis is during a pregnancy, according to the National Health Service in the United Kingdom: [50]

"If you get Toxoplasmosis in the early stages of pregnancy, there is a greater risk of miscarriage, still birth or birth defects," according to the NHS. It's rare for the infection to pass to the baby during early pregnancy, but if it does it can cause serious health problems. In later-stage pregnancy, it is more common for the infection to pass to the baby. For example:

- if you become infected around the time of conception, there is less than a 1 percent chance that your baby will also develop the infection
- if you become infected during the third trimester of your pregnancy (from week 27 until the birth), there is about a 70 percent chance that your baby will also be infected

However, babies infected during later-stage pregnancy are less likely to develop serious health problems. The disease can have devastating consequences in immunodeficient and congenitally infected individuals. Severe Toxoplasmosis, which causes damage to the brain, eyes, or other organs can occur with an acute infection or reactivate from an earlier infection, according to a paper on Toxoplasmosis produced at Midwestern State University in Wichita Falls, Texas.

The CDC advises the usual cautions when handling food, washing hands, utensils, and cutting boards, cooking meat to at least 160 degrees, and avoiding cross contamination. [51]

Toxoplasmosis is a common cause of death in AIDS patients.

People become infected by eating undercooked, contaminated meat, especially pork, lamb, and venison, and eating food contaminated by knives, utensils, cutting boards, and other food contact surfaces that have had association with raw, contaminated meat.

The CDC estimates that 22.5 percent of the population 12 years and older have been infected with Toxoplasma, but few have symptoms because their immune systems usually keep the parasite from causing illness.

Cyclospora

Cyclospora is a parasite that causes an intestinal infection called Cyclosporiasis. In 2013, the Centers for Disease Control and Prevention received data on 631 cases of Cyclosporiasis from 25 states. [52] Forty-nine people were hospitalized. There were no deaths reported from the pathogen.

The CDC investigated a major outbreak of Cyclospora infections in the spring of 1996, after victims ate tainted Guatemalan raspberries.[53] More than 2,500 people in 21 states and two Canadian provinces developed the disease.

Donna Heller, a 54-year-old teacher from Crowley, a small town south of Fort Worth, Texas, says she lost her appetite, eating only a few bites of food, before feeling uncomfortably full and needing to run to the bathroom.[54] She told ABC News, "I had to wait three weeks to find out what was wrong." She added, "It was very frustrating. I found myself in tears a lot of the time."

Ms. Heller had the classic symptoms of the "stomach flu," which invariably turns out to be a foodborne illness; nausea, diarrhea, cramps, and bloating just would not go away. She made several attempts to get an appointment with a doctor, to no avail. Finally, after a trip to a 24-hour clinic and a few days later, a call from the CDC revealed she had contracted a Cyclospora parasite.[55] She told medical investigators that while dieting she had eaten a lot of lettuce in the days prior to the onset of her illness. Ms. Heller became a statistic, one of more than 500 people in 16 states infected in 2013 with the Cyclospora parasite. Health officials in Iowa and Nebraska traced the source to Taylor Farms de Mexico, a part of Taylor Farms in California.[56] But the FDA and CDC did not find the source of the outbreak in the other 14 states.

AROUND THE WORLD

Massive outbreaks of foodborne illnesses obviously are not restricted to the United States. The World Health Organization reported an outbreak of Hepatitis A caused by eating raw, tainted clams that affected nearly 300,000 people in Shanghai, China, in 1988.[57] The clams were harvested from a bay polluted with sewage from a community that had experienced an epidemic of Hepatitis A.

In July 1996, about 7,000 children in Sakai City, Japan, became ill, and some died, in the largest outbreak of E. coli O157:H7.[58] Investigators traced the cause to the consumption of contaminated white radish sprouts served through a centralized school lunch program.

A 1980 outbreak in Spain resulted in the deaths of 800 people and 20,000 others becoming sick, many of whom remained ill more than 10 years later. Investigators traced the cause to a chemical agent present in cooking oil. Toxic Oil Syndrome (TOS) proved to be a new disease, one that is complicated and intriguing from a scientific viewpoint, according to the World Health Organization.[59] Consumption of illicitly refined rapeseed oil caused the problem. Rapeseed oil production varies from feed for animals, vegetable oil for human consumption, and biodiesel as a fuel for standard diesel engines.

In the 1960s, a Japanese outbreak of mercury poisoning sickened more than 200 people who ate highly contaminated fish caught in polluted waters. [60]

Food poisonings can occur in the simplest of foods. Even one of the world's oldest foods, sometimes called manna, can become contaminated. The CDC and WHO reported a 1971 outbreak in Iraq that killed 459 people and hospitalized more than 6,500 with neurological symptoms after eating bread made from mercury-contaminated wheat. [61]

Chapter Eleven

Food Tampering and Food Fraud

FOOD TAMPERING

It's not just the terrorist we need to defend against to prevent or lessen the effects of an attack on our food supplies. Incidents of food tampering are sporadic, yet often are followed by copycat cases. You should always carefully open cartons, packages, bottles, and other containers that do not have a security seal, making sure there are no signs that someone else may have been there before you.

Improvements in packaging make it nearly impossible to tamper with certain products without leaving obvious signs. We've come a long way, but many other problems may be virtually impossible to stop. The ways and means of tampering with food have become creative, imaginative, widely varied, and frightening, as we see in these unrelated cases: [1]

- Members of the Rajneeshee religious cult contaminated salad bars with Salmonella Typhimurium to disrupt a local election in Oregon in 1984. [2] Salmonellosis hit 751 people, hospitalizing 45 of the victims, according to Marc L. Ostfield, senior advisor for bioterrorism, biodefense, and health security at the U.S. Department of State. Ostfield is an expert on protecting our food supply. In 1996, a disgruntled Texas lab worker infected food prepared for coworkers, sickening 12 people with Shigella dysenteria type 2 and hospitalizing four other victims, Ostfield said. [3]
- In May 2003, a supermarket employee in Grand Rapids, Michigan, pleaded guilty to intentionally poisoning 200 pounds of ground beef with Black Leaf 40, an insecticide, which has a main ingredient of nicotine. [4] Police say the suspect wanted to get his supervisor in trouble and eventually was sentenced to nine years in prison and assessed restitution of

$12,000 that he had to pay. The meat was sold in only one store, but that was enough to make 111 people ill. All complained of burning of the mouth, nausea, vomiting, and dizziness. The victims included about three dozen children, a pregnant woman, and an elderly man with heart problems. Emergency room doctors treated one person for atrial fibrillation, according to Ostfield.[5]

- The infamous 1984 Girl Scout Cookie tampering cases spread across at least 16 states.
- Needles and other foreign objects had been placed in boxes of the cookies that were sold door-to-door. More than 800 persons received cuts and puncture wounds, but no critical injuries occurred. Pins and needles reportedly found in cookies probably were inserted by children playing pranks or by publicity-seekers in their own homes, according to Bill Grigg, a spokesman for the FDA, which worked on the investigation with the FBI.[6] The cookie boxes were modified the following year.
- In 1986 the FDA received 140 complaints about broken glass in Gerber's baby food products.[7] The FBI confirmed filing 21 criminal cases, all believed to be private individuals rather than an organized group.

The CDC also focused on food sabotage from other countries' experiences to learn more about this serious worldwide problem. In Great Britain in 1989, a purported blackmailer tried to extort almost $2 million from the manufacturer, H.J. Heinz and Cow & Gate, targeting baby food.[8] Slivers of glass, razor blades, and pins showed up in numerous jars of baby food. Incidents of this alarming strain of crime, which can have devastating consequences for the consumer and the product companies involved, have been less frequent in Britain than in the United States. And Britain has never experienced catastrophic product tampering cases like the one in Chicago in 1982, when seven died after taking doses of Tylenol, a Johnson & Johnson pain reliever, that had been laced with cyanide, or like the one in Japan in 1985, when eight people died after drinking fruit juice contaminated by weed killer, according to the *New York Times*.[9] Yet by almost any standard the British case was dramatic and troubling. Razor blades, pins, caustic soda, and slivers of glass were found in the baby food.[10]

Masked extortionists in Japan in 1984 used cyanide-laced Glico candy as the ransom vehicle in the kidnapping of Katsuhisa Ezaki, president of the Glico Confectionary Company.[11] The suspects asked a ransom of one billion yen and 100 kg of gold bullion. Ezaki escaped three days later. Japanese police found packages of Angel Pie and Morinaga Choco Balls tainted with cyanide. Apparently, no one had purchased any of the contaminated candies. The case remains unsolved. A year later, eight people in Japan died after drinking fruit juice injected with some type of herbicide. Japanese health officials released no further information on the poisonings.[12]

In 2002, nearly 40 people died and more than 200 were hospitalized near Nanjing, China, after the owner of a fast-food outlet poisoned a competitor's breakfast foods with rat poison.[13] A year earlier, 120 people in China were sickened when the owners of a noodle factory reportedly laced their food with rat poison, according to the U.S. Department of State.[14]

A Palestinian militant group, the Arab Revolutionary Army, claimed responsibility in 1978 for the injection of mercury into citrus fruit from Israel to induce panic and disrupt that country's economy.[15] A couple in the Netherlands made the discovery when their four children noticed a strange taste in the Jaffa oranges. The children were treated at a hospital emergency room and authorities opened an investigation. Some of the contaminated fruit showed up in England, Spain, and Germany.

Twenty years later, a possible politically motivated copycat incident involved Chilean grapes and other fruit laced with cyanide and found at the Port of Philadelphia after an annonymous phone tip to the U.S. FDA.[16] The tampering case publicized deplorable living conditions in the Chilean slums.

A drug addict in the United Arab Emirates in 1998 used his access as a nurse to a cardiac intensive care unit to extract fentanyl, a synthetic opioid analgesic 100 times more potent than morphine, for his habit.[17] He replaced the liquid medicine with water for use on the next patient.

The "aquabomber," as he or she was dubbed by police in Italy in 2003, sent more than two dozen people to hospitals after they drank bottled water contaminated with bleach or ammonia injected under the plastic caps.[18] No one claimed responsibility. Similar copycat incidents occurred in 20 other Italian cities.

Sometimes no motive exists in intentional food contamination cases. Australian authorities say a mentally unstable woman from Brisbane used rat poison pellets to contaminate salad bars at Sizzler restaurants in Queensland.[19] The woman made no demands. No serious injuries occurred.

Copycat crimes, always a problem, usually occur after the original crime. One 12-year-old was part of a chain reaction of copycat events at a Fairfax County, Virginia, school in 2007.[20] The seventh-grade student was charged with felony food tampering after school officials found a straight pin in a bowl of applesauce. Three similar crimes followed within a two-week period. A few days later a student found an inch-long piece of a paper clip in a piece of chicken.

Some tampering cases go all the way to trial, conviction, and appeal and often without success on the part of the defendant. In 2011, a 45-year-old Calgary woman, Tatyana Granada, was found guilty of mischief and trespassing for placing needles, pins, nails, and other objects into bread, cheese, and produce at a local co-op that estimated it lost at least $600,000 in business and in costs connected with the investigation.[21] In July 2013 the woman lost her appeal and was ordered to begin serving a three-year prison sentence.

The Canadian Food Inspection Agency has studied food fraud and tampering cases and suggests several reasons for such crime, at least in the minds of the perpetrators, and some signs to look for in possible food tampering:

Reasons

Those who engage in food tampering are usually after something. Their motives can include:

- Publicity
- Extortion for gain
- Mischief or prank
- Revenge
- Reasons known only to the perpetrator
- Terrorism

Signs of food tampering

- Packaging that has been opened and resealed
- Products that have damaged or missing safety seals or tamper-evident seals
- Products or packaging that is cut, torn, punctured, or discolored
- Products that are dirty or damaged
- Products with strange odor or flavor
- Cans or jars with signs of leakage, spillage, or corrosion
- Vacuum-packed products with no vacuum seal
- Packaging that has been altered, including labels, product lot codes, and other identifying information
- The presence of a foreign object or non-food item in the product

Steps you should take

- Call 9-1-1 and report the incident.
- Do not eat the product, obviously. If you are experiencing symptoms, seek immediate medical intervention.
- Do not change the product and its wrapping or carton in any way.
- Write down information as to where and when you purchased the product.
- In the United States, call the FDA 24-hour emergency number at 866-300-4374 or 301-796-8240; in Canada, call the Canadian Food Inspection Agency at 800-442-2342.

FOOD FRAUD

Food fraud differs from food tampering in that the fraud usually does not involve actions that could make you sick. Some product switching or substitutions could affect those with various food allergies. Olive oil heads the most prevalent food frauds, followed by milk, honey, saffron, orange juice, coffee, and apple juice.

Fraud conducted for economic gain by food producers and manufacturers caught the attention of industry, governments, and standards-setting organizations. Food fraud, differing greatly from agroterrorism, is defined as encompassing the deliberate substitution, addition, or tampering of food for economic gain. The difference is economic gains versus terrorism.

Horse meat labeled as beef sold throughout Europe created a major, ongoing scandal.[22] Several Chinese were arrested in 2012 for selling rat meat labeled as lamb.[23] Over the years, investigators found a myriad of adulterants in milk, including melamine, maltodextrin, formaldehyde, hydrogen peroxide, machine oil, cow tallow, palm oil, urea, whey, cane sugar, lactose, detergent, caustic soda, hydrolyzed leather, sodium dodecylbenzene sulfonate, gardenia yellow dye, and pork lard, according to the U.S. Pharmacopeial Convention's Food Fraud Database. Melamine, an organic base and trimer of cyanamide, contains 67 percent nitrogen by mass with fire-retardant properties and has been implicated with contaminants in Chinese protein adulterations. Dodecylbenzene sulfonate is a major component of laundry soap.

The *New York Times* in June 2013 published a report on counterfeit food and how the problem is spreading. In the article, reporters Stephen Castle and Doreen Carvajal wrote that "investigators have uncovered thousands of frauds, raising fresh questions about regulatory oversight as criminals offer bargain-hunting shoppers cheap versions of everyday products, including counterfeit chocolate and adulterated olive oil, Jacob's Creek wine, and even Bollinger Champagne. As the horsemeat scandal showed, even legitimate companies can be overtaken by the murky world of food fraud."[24]

Accounts of food fraud incidents collected from 1980 to 2010 have been included in the eighth edition of the U.S. Pharmacopeial Convention's Food Chemicals Codex and include 1,305 records from 677 references.[25] Olive oil, milk, honey, and saffron were the most common targets for adulteration reported in scholarly journals, and potentially harmful issues identified include spices diluted with lead chromate and lead tetraoxide, substitution of Chinese star anise with toxic Japanese star anise, and melamine adulteration of high-protein foods, according to the Codex.

The 2007 tainted cheese conspiracy triggered criminal actions against unscrupulous food companies in Chicago.[26] Five years after officials discovered a scheme to ship 110,000 pounds of contaminated cheese adulterated with Salmonella and E. coli, a federal grand jury handed up a six-count indictment against three men and one woman who are awaiting trial. The indictments alleged that mold and fungus had been scraped off the cheese and then sold to customers.

Bottles labeled "Extra Virgin Olive Oil" turned out to be bottles of corn oil, sunflower oil, or soybean oil. In China, secondhand oil, referred to on the street as gutter oil, was sold as olive oil. [27]

Investigators found many spices illegally adulterated. [28] Lead tetraoxide was substituted for paprika; leaves from sumac and citrus or coffee husks were substituted for oregano; and dung powder was illegally sold under the name coriander. The substitutions go on and on: starch for turmeric powder; dehydrated red beets for chili powder; basic red 46 dye for sumac spice; flowers from marigold for the expensive saffron; and lead chromate–adulterated turmeric.

Vietnamese catfish were passed off as grouper, pacific dog snapper was substituted for red snapper, and all too often Atlantic or farm-raised salmon replaced Pacific or wild-caught salmon.

In addition to outright criminal fraud in some of the food purchased, deceptive labeling cropped up in many sections of supermarkets. The consumer advocacy group Center for Science in the Public Interest (CSPI) for decades exposed questionable and outright false advertising of foods. [29]

CSPI filed complaints with the FDA about egregiously mislabeled foods—for example,"blueberry" waffles with no blueberries or "strawberry" yogurt for kids with no strawberries. Food manufacturers see the FDA's inaction on such products as a signal to make even more deceptive claims.

During the past 10 years, CSPI aggressively attacked the problem of false or misleading advertising with lawsuits and pressures on Congress and food manufacturing companies. "Food manufacturers are shamelessly tricking consumers who are trying to eat more fruits, vegetables, and whole grains," said CSPI director of legal affairs Bruce Silverglade. [30] "Too many processed foods contain only token amounts of the healthful ingredients highlighted on labels and are typically loaded with fats, refined sugars, refined flour, and salt, in various combinations," he said.

At a news conference in Washington with Representative Rosa DeLauro (D-CT) and Connecticut attorney general Richard Blumenthal (now Senator Blumenthal), Silverglade said that the FDA should immediately stop the practice of misleading food labels, including those for the following:

- Gerber Graduates for Toddlers Fruit Juice Snacks. The package is decorated with pictures of oranges, cherries, and strawberries, but the leading ingredients are corn syrup and sugar. "You can guess why Gerber doesn't call these things Corn Syrup Snacks—no parent would buy them," says Silverglade. "This is candy, not fruit juice."

- Betty Crocker Super Moist Carrot Cake Mix. The box depicts what appears to be pieces of carrot, but the only carrot ingredient is "carrot powder," which is the 19th ingredient listed, behind artificial color, salt, and dicalcium phosphate.
- Smucker's Simply 100% Fruit. The strawberry version of this "100% fruit" spread contains 30 percent strawberries; the blueberry version contains only 43 percent blueberries. Both have more fruit syrup that comes not from berries but from less expensive apple, pineapple, or pear juice concentrate.
- Kellogg's Eggo Nutri-Grain Pancakes. The label boasts that these pancakes are "Made with Whole Wheat and Whole Grain," but the pancakes are made primarily with white flour and have more high-fructose corn syrup than whole wheat or other whole grain. CSPI says that foods labeled "whole grain" should have whole grain flour as their flour constituent, as is the requirement for whole wheat bread.
- General Mills Yoplait Light Fat Free Yogurt. The label claims that if consumers eat three servings of milk, cheese, or yogurt daily it helps to burn more fat and helps dieters lose weight. However, the U.S. government's Dietary Guidelines Advisory Committee has called the evidence on dairy products and weight loss inconclusive.
- Quaker Oats Pasta Roni. The label boasts "white cheddar & broccoli" in large letters and displays a picture of pasta with pieces of broccoli. Although broccoli appears on the fourth line of a 14-line ingredient list, there are only small specks of broccoli in the actual package.

Of 9,000 employees, the FDA has the equivalent of only four full-time headquarters staff enforcing food-labeling laws, a staffing level that CSPI says has proven to be completely incapable of ensuring honest labels on the $500 billion worth of FDA-regulated foods. Nevertheless, even with those few staffers, CSPI says the agency could still be much more aggressive in policing misleading labels.[31]

Chapter Twelve

Foods We Eat, Others Won't

If our food is as safe as it can be made, as our government claims, why do other countries around the world consider many of the foods we eat so dangerous that they ban them from reaching their consumers? We unknowingly shove questionable additives and chemicals down our throats, while consumers in other countries have been afforded necessary protection by their governments, which forbid any import, manufacture, or production of these foods and additives. The list of some of these food additives is enlightening and frightening.

Arsenic

Arsenic gained its notoriety in part because in movies it became the poison of choice to commit murder. Arsenic added to poultry feed to more quickly fatten the birds speeds their trip to the slaughterhouse, putting more dollars in the pockets of chicken and turkey processors. Organically raised chickens contain considerably less arsenic.[1] New studies increasingly link the arsenic in poultry feed to serious human health problems.

"FDA could easily and immediately fix the problem, but instead puts its head in the sand," according to Paige Tomaselli, senior staff attorney with the Center for Food Safety (CFS).[2] This consumer advocacy group, along with the Institute for Agriculture and Trade Policy (IATP) and seven other public health and environmental groups, sued the FDA, calling for a response from the federal government on the groups' three-year-old petition calling for a ban on arsenic in feed for food animals. The Center for Food Safety picked up the issue with a lengthy article supporting the lawsuit. "FDA leadership is asleep at the switch, if not turning a blind eye to public health," said David Wallinga, MD, a physician with the IATP. "Seven years ago,

IATP blew the whistle on FDA's indifference to arsenic being needlessly fed to chickens and turkeys. More than a decade ago, we sounded the alarm on how the FDA let the routine feeding of drugs to chickens and turkeys help ensure that Americans would eat meat often contaminated with bacteria resistant to multiple antibiotics," according to Wallinga.[3]

The United States fails to ban arsenic on the federal level, so the state of Maryland took care of the problem and wisely banned arsenic in January 2013.[4] A ban on arsenic applies in all 28 countries comprising the European Union.

Bread and Frozen Dinners with Azodicarbonamide

Using azodicarbonamide in the "Lion City" is a criminal offense.[5,6] Yes, if you ran a restaurant in Singapore and used the chemical azodicarbonamide in food you're serving, you could face up to 15 years in prison and a $500,000 fine.[7] As a food additive, the product serves as a bleaching agent in cereal flour. Most frozen bread products, some frozen fried potatoes, and Hungry Man frozen dinners contain the chemical, which is also used to make rubber yoga mats.

Azodicarbonamide can bleach flour, and it can be used to put the foam in plastics. The heat in the environment makes the difference in safe or unsafe conditions. The ingredient can cause asthma and skin problems.

Subway sandwich shops in the United Kingdom, all European Union countries, and Australia do not use azodicarbonamide.[8] But, Subway for years had been using it in at least eight of its breads in stores in the United States until February 2014. The publicity about the dangers of azodicarbonamide forced Subway to stop using the additive.[9]

U.S. senator Charles Schumer (D-NY) announced a major push for the FDA to ban azodicarbonamide from all foods because he had found that the additive is "suspected to be a carcinogen."[10] Schumer went on to point out, as was just mentioned, that the 28 countries making up the European Union, along with Australia, have banned azodicarbonamide while the U.S. FDA currently approves it.[11] "Other fast-food chains are known to use this chemical in their bread products as well, including McDonald's, Starbucks, Arby's, Wendy's, Burger King, Kentucky Fried Chicken, and various grocery store chains and other restaurants," Schumer's news release stated. Singapore also bans azodicarbonamide in foods.[12]

According to the Federal Registry, the FDA approves the use of azodicarbonamide in bread but appears to stick its head in the sand by indicating it doesn't know this additive is currently used in the United States.[13] Here's what the Everything Added to Food in the United States (EAFUS) database has to say about azodicarbonamide: "Although listed as added to food, there is no current reported use of the substance, and, therefore, although toxicology information may be available in PAFA (Priority-Based Assessment of Food Additives), it is not being updated."[14]

The United Kingdom, most European countries, Australia, and Singapore have banned the use of azodicarbonamide.

Kraft Macaroni & Cheese and Other Foods with Food Coloring

Two concerned and enterprising women from North Carolina, worried about the health of their children because of yellow dye 5 and yellow dye 6 in Kraft Macaroni & Cheese, did some investigating on their own.[15] To the amazement of Lisa Leake and Vani Hari, their probing turned up data regarding Kraft's production of the same Macaroni & Cheese for sale in the United Kingdom free of all dyes. Why? The UK has stricter laws and forbids most dyes. But the women's surprise and disappointment goes further. For its UK customers, Kraft uses natural beta carotene and paprika to make virtually the same color as the yellow dyes. Kraft doesn't offer the healthier product to American consumers.[16]

The women told ABC News in March 2013, "The yellow dye serves only 'aesthetic purposes.' We worry that food colorings have been associated with hyperactivity in children, allergies, migraine and, because yellow dyes are petroleum-based, may be cancer-causing." The synthetic yellow dye is known as tartrazine.[17]

A 1994 study at the University of Melbourne suggested that children previously identified as hyperactive may exhibit an increase in irritability, restlessness, and sleep disturbance after ingesting tartrazine. Norway, Austria, and Germany banned tartrazine. The European Union overturned the ban and Germany had to reverse its decision.

"The British Food Standards Agency has advised parents to consider eliminating artificial food colors from the diet, and the European Union has called for eliminating six colors or listing on the label the warning that '[the color] may have an adverse effect on activity and attention in children,'" according to *Environmental Health Perspectives*, a publication of the U.S. National Library of Medicine.[18] The FDA only requires a designation on the products that contain tartrazine or yellow dye. "Food dyes—used in everything from M&Ms to Manischewitz Matzo Balls to Kraft salad dressings—pose risks of cancer, hyperactivity in children, and allergies, and should be banned," according to a news report by the Center for Science in the Public Interest.[19] The extremely knowledgeable food safety expert Michael Jacobson, executive director of the CSPI, in June 2010 called for the FDA to ban yellow #5. "These synthetic chemicals do absolutely nothing to improve the nutritional quality or safety of foods, but trigger behavior problems in children and, possibly, cancer in anybody," he said.[20] Jacobson added that a ban on the dyes would force industry to color foods with real food ingredients, not toxic petrochemicals. Per capita consumption of dyes has increased five-fold since the mid-1950s.

An East Bridgewater, Massachusetts, woman, Heather Brodie Perry, petitioned the FDA, citing numerous concerns and fears she had with yellow #5, and called for a delisting or ban on the additive.[21] She stated reasons why she believed FDA's standards of safety are not met with yellow #5. In the petition Ms. Perry related her experience with the additive. "On December 18, 1999 my 20-month-old son had a cold, so as a treat I gave him a cup of commercially prepared eggnog. Rapidly, he was overtaken by an asthma attack so severe he nearly died. Our local hospital, unable to handle the emergency, called in a team of doctors from Children's Hospital in Boston. They treated Ryan with a drug typically reserved for adults with COPD. Later, we discovered the cause of this reaction was the artificial coloring in the eggnog."

Another reason Ms. Perry believes that the approval of yellow #5 should be revoked focuses on the Delaney Clause, part of federal law that restricts the FDA from approving "for use in food any chemical additive found to induce cancer in man, or, after tests, found to induce cancer in animals."[22] "The Delaney Clause establishes a zero cancer risk for food additives. Tartrazine has not been shown to cause cancer. But one of the chemicals used in making tartrazine, benzidine, is a carcinogen. Federal law mandates that the level of benzidine in tartrazine be less than one part per billion but studies in the journal *Food Additives Contamination* have shown that in many cases this level is more than 200 parts per billion," Ms. Perry said.

Yellow #5 is banned in Norway, Finland, Austria, France, and the United Kingdom.[23]

Brominated Vegetable Oil (BVO)

Bromine vapors can be toxic, and consuming bromine directly can be compared to consuming chlorine, according to some scientists. Bromine is described as a corrosive gas, and, according to Duke University professor Derek Lowe, speaking with ABC News, "When a bromine atom is bonded to a carbon, as it is in BVO, it's no longer bromine-the-pure-element, any more than the chlorine in table salt is the World War I poison gas, or the phosphorus in your DNA is the burning white phosphorus found in military tracer shells."[24]

Brominated vegetable oil is banned in more than 100 European countries and in Japan.

Recombinant Bovine Growth Hormone (rBGH)

While the evidence continues to stack up against the use of rBGH, the "FDA stubbornly sticks to its position that milk from rBGH-treated cows is no different than milk from untreated cows . . . this is just plain false and is not supported by science," according to the website of Dr. Joseph M. Mercola, DO.[25] The bovine growth hormone increases milk production in dairy cattle while converting normal tissue cells into cancerous ones, increasing colorectal, prostate, and breast cancer risks.[26] In 1999, the United Nations Safety Agency ruled unanimously not to endorse or set safety standards for rBGH milk, which has effectively resulted in an international ban on U.S. milk. Non-organic dairy farms frequently have rBGH-injected cows that suffer at least 16 different adverse health conditions, including very high rates of mastitis, which contaminates milk with pus and antibiotics.[27] In 2010, a petition to FDA commissioner Margaret Hamburg calling for a dairy industry ban of rBGH was rejected, and the FDA continued its unpopular position that rBGH-treated milk is no different than milk from untreated cows.[28] What to do now? Look for products labeled "rBGH-free."

Australia, New Zealand, Canada, Japan, Israel, and the 28 European Union countries banned rBGH because of the dangerous impacts on both human and animal health.

Potassium Bromate in Wraps, Rolls, Bread Crumbs, and Bagel Chips

Potassium bromate is considered throughout most of the world as a potential cause of cancer in humans. It's also known to damage the nervous system. In the United States, potassium bromate is used to strengthen dough in bread making for things like wraps, rolls, bread crumbs, bagels, and bagel chips. It's also an additive to BVO. Some scientists say only negligible residues of potassium bromate remain after baking. California requires a cancer warning label on products if potassium bromate has been added.[29] Potassium bromate is banned in the 28 nations of the European Union, Canada, China, Sri Lanka, Nigeria, Brazil, and Peru.

Cereal, Nuts, Meat, and Other Foods with BHA

Butylated hydroxyanisole (BHA) is used primarily as an antioxidant and preservative in food, food packaging, animal feed, and cosmetics and in rubber and petroleum products. The CSPI reports that some studies demonstrate that "butylated hydroxyanisole (BHA), found in cereals, chewing gum, potato chips and vegetable oil, causes cancer in rats, mice, and hamsters." Those cancer studies are controversial because the cancers they found occurred in the forestomach, an organ that humans do not have. However, a chemical that causes cancer in at least one organ in three different species indicates that it might be carcinogenic in humans.[30] That is why the U.S. Department of Health and Human Services considers BHA to be "reasonably anticipated to be a human carcinogen." Nevertheless, the FDA still permits BHA to be used as a preservative in foods. This synthetic chemical can be replaced by safer chemicals (e.g., vitamin E), can be used with safer processes (e.g., packing foods under nitrogen instead of air), or can simply be left out (many brands of oily foods, such as potato chips, don't use any antioxidant).

The State of California lists butylated hydroxyanisole as a possible carcinogen. Japan, England, and many other European countries have banned BHA.

Astaxanthin

Synthetic astaxanthin is not manufactured for human consumption.[31] It is synthesized from petrochemicals and sold as feed for chickens, shrimp, crabs, and salmon. If you eat farm-raised salmon, you're receiving synthetic astaxanthin that is not approved as a human food or a supplement ingredient in food nor is FDA approved as generally recognized as safe (GRAS).

On the other hand, natural astaxanthin is biosynthesized and serves as a powerful health benefit for humans.

Farm-raised fish or shellfish of any type that are fed synthetic astaxanthin made from petrochemicals have not been approved for human consumption. Farmed salmon fed astaxanthin are banned in Australia and New Zealand.

Hawaiian Papaya with Genetically Modified Organisms (GMOs)

GMO Hawaiian papayas are banned in all European Union countries because it may have to do with research showing that animals fed other genetically engineered foods, like soy and corn, are prone to intestinal and organ damage, tumors, birth defects, premature death, and near complete sterility by the third generation.[32] The EU awaits additional research on GMO papayas.

Meat with Ractopamine

Questionable testing of meat containing ractopamine should be enough to ban the additive, but instead the FDA, siding with the producers, wants to simply limit its use. The manufacturers of the drug-like growth additive have enjoyed stealth use in the U.S. food supply for more than a decade, despite being banned almost everywhere else. Ractopamine as brand name Paylean® is fed to pigs; as Optaflexx®, it fattens cattle; and turkeys feast on Topmax® to enable the animals to gain weight quicker.[33] Ractopamine in meat is banned in 160 countries across Europe and in Russia, Japan, mainland China, and the Republic of China (Taiwan). (Ractopamine is discussed more fully in chapter 6.)

Fat-Free Chips with Olestra or Olean

When you take the worst of the unhealthiest foods and make it even more unhealthy, there's something seriously wrong with our diet. In an effort to make the high-fat-content potato chip a little less fattening, some manufacturers have produced chips with lower fat content but using a fat substitute called olestra. The lowly potato chip is victimized by olestra, sometimes referred to as olean.[34] This additive causes a depletion of fat-soluble carotenoid and much needed vitamins. Olestra also deprives us of micronutrients that we should be getting.

Lay's WOW chips and Ruffles Light are the only brands of potato chips containing olestra, which is banned in the U.K. and Canada.[35]

American children are exposed to approximately 40,000 food advertisements per year, 72 percent of which are for candy, cereal, and fast food.[36] Empirical studies, including recent reviews by the American Psychological Association and the Institute of Medicine (IOM), show that advertisements achieve their intended effects on children—that is, they shape product preferences and eating habits. Moreover, children younger than eight years of age are generally unable to understand the persuasive intent of advertising and to view it critically.

Chapter Thirteen

Unwelcome Critters in Our Foods

I found some surprising, unwanted, and disconcerting animal and mineral items in our food. But it's no problem; it's naturally occurring, says the U.S. FDA. The FDA is well aware of these disgusting items but says it's economically impossible to completely correct. [1] While the FDA contends that maggots, rodent hairs, some excrement, and scores of other elements won't hurt us, some chemicals found in these "ingredients" present a serious potential for brain damage, cancer, and other critical illnesses. [2]

Biosolids

Biosolids, a deceptively clean-sounding name for human waste that's spread on some of our food crops as fertilizer, raise serious questions about its use. Long known as "night soil," the human waste is now treated and the resulting sludge acts as fertilizer and makes crops grow faster, putting more money in producers' pockets. Opponents say the sludge cannot be considered safe and people near the fields are getting sick. [3]

A 2002 study found that people living within about a mile of biosolids application sites suffered skin rashes and burning of the eyes, throat, and lungs. "A prevalence of Staphylococcus Aureus infections of the skin and respiratory tract was found. Approximately one in four of 54 individuals were infected and two died in the Robesonia area of Pennsylvania." One death was attributed to pneumonia; the other to septicemia, more commonly called blood poisoning. [4]

Recycling companies obtain the biosolids from municipal wastewater treatment plants after filtering and treatment of the water is performed according to federal regulations. [5] The sludge also contains pharmaceuticals, medical wastes, and all the things that corporations and residents flush down the drain.

Whole Foods Markets agreed in early 2014 to stop selling produce grown in sewage sludge biosolids due to its toxic contents of hazardous chemicals.[6] The U.S. Clean Water Act requires the EPA to identify and regulate toxic pollutants that may be present in biosolids at levels of concern for public health and the environment. The sampling of biosolids from 74 randomly selected sites produced 145 analytes or chemical substances including 28 metals, 4 polycyclic aromatic hydrocarbons, 11 flame retardants, 72 pharmaceuticals, and 25 steroids and hormones.

OTHER PRODUCTS THE FDA ALLOWS IN
OUR FOODS AND WHY

A March 2012 report by the *Huffington Post* vividly explored "crushed cochineal beetles in your favorite strawberry-flavored Starbucks drinks, plus meat glue and ammonia in ground beef.[7] The details surprised and shocked most consumers." But perhaps more shocking is a list of several hundred products allowed by the FDA to contain little critters, along with some excrement from mice and other surprises.

Let this next statement sink in for a moment. It comes from the U.S. FDA: "The FDA set these action levels because it is not economical or practical to grow and process certain foods to the point that they contain no insect fragments and other defects." Is that the government's only defense? I don't believe consumers are going to buy it. How about making a more serious effort to at least reduce the allowable number of "defects"? The government calls them "natural or unavoidable defects in foods for human use that present no health hazard." So it's safe for more than one hundred different foods we eat to contain a certain amount of maggots, rodent hairs, fly eggs, larvae, mold, and rot. It's the law. These foods "pose no inherent hazard to health," according to the FDA.

Here are examples of some of the foods the FDA allows to have "defects" and the maximum amount of filth that we really don't want to eat:

- Apple butter: four or more rodent hairs per 100 grams of product
- Asparagus, canned or frozen: 10 percent by count of spears or pieces infested with six or more attached asparagus beetle eggs and/or sacs
- Bay leaves: mold on average of 5 percent or more pieces by weight
- Berries, canned and frozen: average of four or more larvae per 500 grams
- Broccoli, frozen: average of 60 or more aphids and/or thrips and/or mites per 100 grams

- Brussels sprouts, frozen: average of 30 or more aphids and/or thrips per 100 grams
- Cinnamon, ground: average of 400 or more insect fragments per 50 grams; average of 11 or more rodent hairs per 50 grams
- Cherries, fresh or frozen: average of 7 percent or more pieces rejected due to rot; average of 4 percent or more pieces rejected due to insects other than maggots
- Cherries, maraschino: average of 5 percent or more pieces rejected due to maggots
- Chocolate and chocolate liquor: average of 60 or more insect fragments per 100 grams when six 100-gram subsamples are examined, or 90 or more insect fragments in any one subsample; average of one or more rodent hairs per 100 grams in six 100-gram subsamples examined or three or more rodent hairs in any one subsample
- Citrus fruit juices: five or more drosophila and other fly eggs per 250 milliliters or one or more maggots per 250 milliliters
- Cocoa beans: more than 4 percent of beans by count insect infested
- Coffee beans, green: average of 10 percent or more by count insect-infested or insect-damaged
- Corn, sweet, canned: two or more 3-millimeter or longer larvae, cast skins, or larval or cast skin fragments of corn ear worms or corn borer, with aggregate length of such larvae, cast skins, or larval or cast skin fragments exceeding 12 millimeters in 24 pounds (24 No. 303 cans or equivalent)
- Cornmeal: average of one or more rodent hairs per 25 grams
- Eggs, frozen: two or more cans decomposed and at least two subsamples from decomposed cans with direct microscopic counts of five million or more bacteria per gram
- Fennel seed: 20 percent or more of subsamples with mammalian excreta
- Fish (bluefin and other freshwater herring): 60 parasitic cysts per 100 fish or 100 pounds of fish averaging over one pound, provided that 20 percent of the fish examined are infested
- Macaroni and noodle products: average of 225 insect fragments or more per 225 grams in six or more subsamples; average of 4.5 rodent hairs or more per 225 grams in six or more samples
- Mushrooms, canned and dried: average of over 20 or more maggots of any size per 100 grams of drained mushrooms and proportionate liquid or 15 grams of dried mushrooms; average of 75 mites per 100 grams drained mushrooms and proportionate liquid or 15 grams of dried mushrooms
- Oregano, ground: average of 1,250 or more insects per 10 grams; average of five or more rodent hairs per 10 grams
- Paprika, ground: average mold count more than 20 percent; average of more than 75 insect fragments per 25 grams; average of more than 11 rodent hairs per 25 grams

- Peaches, canned and frozen: average of 3 percent or more fruit by count wormy or moldy; in 12 one-pound cans, one or more larvae and/or larval fragments whose aggregate length exceeds 5 millimeters
- Peanut butter: average of 30 or more insect fragments per 100 grams; average of one or more rodent hairs per 100 grams; gritty taste and water-insoluble inorganic residue more than 25 milligrams per 100 grams
- Pepper, ground: average of 475 or more insect fragments per 50 grams; average of two or more rodent hairs per 50 grams
- Popcorn: one or more rodent excreta pellets in one or more subsamples and one or more rodent hairs in two or more other subsamples or two or more rodent hairs per pound and rodent hair in 50 percent or more of the subsamples or 20 or more gnawed grains per pound and rodent hair in 50 percent or more of the subsamples
- Raisins, golden: 10 or more whole or equivalent insects and 35 drosophila eggs per 8 ounces
- Sauerkraut: average of more than 50 thrips per 100 grams
- Sesame seeds: average of 5 percent or more seeds by weight insect infested or damaged; average of 5 percent or more seeds by weight decomposed; average of 5 milligrams or more mammalian excreta; average of 0.5 percent or more foreign matter by weight
- Thyme, ground: average of 925 or more insect fragments per 10 grams; average of two or more rodent hairs per 10 grams
- Tomatoes, canned: average of 10 or more drosophila fly eggs per 500 grams or 5 or more fly eggs and one or more maggots per 500 grams or two or more maggots per 500 grams; pizza sauce and other tomato sauces: average mold count in six subsamples 34 percent or more; counts of all subsamples are more than 30 percent
- Wheat: average of 32 or more insect-damaged kernels per 100 grams; average of 9 milligrams or more rodent excreta pellets and/or pellet fragments per kilogram

The FDA appears rather defensive in its responses to some obvious concerns that have flooded the agency's offices in Washington. The FDA set these action levels claiming that it is economically impractical to grow, harvest, or process raw products that are totally free of nonhazardous, naturally occurring, unavoidable defects. Products harmful to consumers are subject to regulatory action whether or not they exceed the action levels.

"It is incorrect to assume that because the FDA has an established defect action level for a food commodity, the food manufacturer need only stay just below that level. The defect levels do not represent an average of the defects that occur in any of the products—the averages are actually much lower. The levels represent limits at which FDA will regard the food product adulterated and subject to enforcement action."[8]

The FDA states on its website that pesticides are not the alternative to preventing food defects. And I certainly agree with that statement. But what are the alternatives to reducing these levels? Perhaps food production methods can be streamlined to eliminate at least some of the filth and extraneous materials. Any move in that direction would be costly, and all the expenses would be passed along to consumers. But usually the FDA and USDA want no part of placing more burdens on businesses while it neglects the needs of consumers.

The FDA continues to exhibit actions and decisions that favor big business rather than look out for the health and safety of consumers. The agency lacks enough funding to hire much-needed inspectors. It is probably not a priority for the FDA to look through any of our food searching for rodent hairs, mites, or maggots when it has bigger problems with antibiotic use and bad slaughtering practices.

What is commonly called "Agent Orange corn," a genetically engineered product, received the feds' green light for production despite having received 45,000 public comments opposing the product and only 23 comments in favor of it. The corn resists the poisonous herbicide 2,4-D, the key ingredient in Agent Orange, which was used during the Vietnam War to defoliate forests and crops, causing serious medical conditions to persons nearby.

So we live with what we've got and with what we're eating until the FDA is forced to decide to make it better.

Chapter Fourteen

GMOs — Genetically Modified Organisms

It was the Christmas holiday 2011. Washington was experiencing warmer than usual weather for December, but things heated up even more over at the U.S. Department of Agriculture, where a well-kept secret plan was about to be quietly put into action.[1] On Tuesday, December 27, 2011, while many lawmakers were still enjoying the Christmas holiday and New Year's vacation, the government gave preliminary approval to a shocking new method for growing corn.[2] The USDA okayed Dow Chemical's genetically engineered (GE) corn, which uses the highly toxic Agent Orange, with its 2,4-D compound, a chemical defoliant used by the United States in Vietnam on the dense fields. The compound 2,4-D can cause serious medical conditions, including birth defects, cancer, and liver disease when humans come in contact with the herbicide. Dow Chemical's genetically engineered version of corn will cause a major increase in the use of 2,4-D, if Dow's unprecedented request to the USDA gains a final approval.[3] Also pending is the U.S. Environmental Protection Agency's decision on a request by Dow Chemical to increase the use of toxic 2,4-D on Dow's Agent Orange crops.[4]

Several months prior to the vote, the USDA had heard from more than 45,000 people and organizations opposed to the company's approval petition on GE corn, and the agency only received 23 comments in support. The opposition comments included a letter with 6,335 signatures, more than 16,000 similar comments from a write-in campaign, and a consolidated document of 22,500 comments.[5] But the preliminary approval slid right through.

Crops that have been modified in unnatural ways through their DNA or have a foreign gene inserted to increase productivity are known as genetically modified organisms (GMOs) and are often referred to as "Frankenfoods," especially in Europe.[6]

Here's a little-publicized fact about GMOs: About 65 percent of processed foods on U.S. grocery shelves have genetically modified ingredients, according to WebMD.[7] Rapeseed oil, maize, and soybeans are the most common genetically modified foods. An article in WebMD suggests that foods made with field corn or high-fructose corn syrup—such as many breakfast cereals, snack foods, cottonseed, and canola-based foods—could likely have genetically modified ingredients.

Consumers simply want labeling of foods containing GMOs so they know what they are buying and eating. But the United States does not require labeling of GMO foods, also often called genetically engineered (GE) foods. Most European countries, along with China and Japan, require all or most GMO foods to be labeled accordingly.[8] In late 2012, Kenya banned all genetically modified food imports.[9]

One of the best definitions I found for "genetically engineered" organisms was from the Biotechnology Project of the Center for Science in the Public Interest:

> When scientists genetically engineer a plant or animal, they remove a gene from one organism (or a specific variety of an organism) and transfer that gene to a different organism (or different variety) using recombinant DNA methods. The new gene becomes integrated into every cell of the organism and is inherited by the organism's offspring. In most cases, the new gene produces a new protein, which then provides the organism with some useful trait.[10]

With genetic engineering, any gene from any organism can be transferred to a different organism. This allows the DNA from a bacterium such as Bacillus thuringiensis, which is a pesticide, to be transferred into a corn or cotton plant, according to CSPI. A CSPI report, "Plugging Holes in the Biotech Safety Net," found that the FDA's oversight of GE food safety is not as rigorous or as independent as it should be, and that the FDA often does not get all of the data it needs to perform a fully informed safety review.[11]

The report leaves open many questions and omissions that the FDA failed to pursue. When the FDA requested additional information to conduct a complete and thorough safety assessment, 50 percent of the time the GE food developer did not comply with that request. In those cases, the FDA had little choice but to complete its evaluation without the desired information.

In three submissions, the data summaries contained obvious errors that were not identified by the FDA during its review process. The submissions did not evaluate some potentially deleterious compounds, such as scientifically recognized toxicants in tomatoes or anti-nutrients that are being added to corn.[12] In addition, allergenicity testing was not always performed using the best tests available.

The data summaries reviewed by the FDA often lacked sufficient detail, such as necessary statistical analyses needed for an adequate safety evaluation. The FDA did not receive adequate data that the transgene and transgenic proteins were unaltered in the GE plant. Safety tests, such as for allergencity, used forms of the protein that may differ from the GE protein found in the transgenic plant. The FDA did not generate its own safety assessment but merely summarized for the public the developer's food-safety analysis.[13]

According to the Center for Science in the Public Interest, to improve the FDA's oversight of GE food crops and the public's confidence in GE foods, the FDA, or Congress where appropriate, should make the following changes:[14]

- Congress should provide the FDA with legal authority for mandatory review and safety approval of GE crops, including the authority to require any data it deems necessary to conduct a thorough food-safety assessment.
- The FDA should develop detailed safety standards and testing guidelines.
- The FDA should require developers to submit not summaries of data, but complete details about their testing methods, the actual data from safety tests, and statistical analyses of those data.
- The FDA should establish an approval process, which is transparent and provides the public with an opportunity to comment on submissions.
- The FDA should perform and make available to the public detailed assessments of commercialized GE crops.
- The FDA should reassess the safety of commercialized GE crops if new safety concerns are recognized or new tests become available.

The CSPI report concluded, "The enormous potential benefits from GE crops and foods will be fully realized only if the FDA's regulatory system is significantly upgraded and enhanced. The changes we have recommended would cost little, but yield big dividends."

Benefits versus Risks

The potential benefits from GMO foods are numerous. Such food could help alleviate starvation in many nations. In the United States, GMOs mean economic gain for the producers. Potential benefits from GE crops include:

- Crops more resistant to weeds and pests
- Bigger yields and more efficient use of land
- Less use of herbicides and pesticides
- Foods with better texture, flavor, and nutritional value
- Foods with long shelf life
- Drought tolerance
- A sustainable way to feed the world[15]

WebMD lists these risks from GMO food and crops: [16]

- Introducing allergens and toxins to food
- Antibiotic resistance
- Adversely changing the nutrient content of a crop
- Creation of "super" weeds and other environmental risks

The *Huffington Post* published an article in September 2013 by Edison de Mello,titled "What's the Big Deal about Genetically-Modified Organisms?" [17] De Mello is also founder and CEO of the Akasha Center for Integrative Medicine and Akasha Naturals. Dr. de Mello begins the article by pointing to 40 industrialized countries, including all of the European Union, that require labeling of GMO foods. He then reminds us, "Nestle, Kraft and Hershey, the ones pouring millions of dollars into defeating the issue at the California polls, do not use GMOs in the European food market." [18]

Are GMO foods safe? "To brush off precaution on the convenient argument that there is not enough evidence to prove that GM food is indeed harmful is sheer irresponsibility. It certainly is a lame excuse to offer in the event that GM foods are indeed proven to contain health hazards," Dr. de Mello writes. [19]

The article points out that the American Academy of Environmental Medicine (AAEM) has warned that genetically modified food poses a serious threat to human health. [20] "Several animal studies indicate serious health risks associated with GM food consumption including infertility, immune dysregulation, accelerated aging, dysregulation of genes associated with cholesterol synthesis, insulin regulation, cell signaling, and protein formation, and changes in the liver, kidney, spleen, and gastrointestinal system," according to AAEM.

Dr. de Mello also referred to a condition called Morgellons disease, which causes crawling, stinging, and biting sensations and lesions of the skin. He says tests on Morgellons patients prove an association with GMO foods. "The Centers for Disease Control and Prevention classified Morgellons disease as being of unknown origin," he said. I found that the CDC no longer pursues a study of Morgellons and considers the condition an "unexplained dermopathy." [21]

Several thousand grocery stores vowed in the summer of 2013 to not sell genetically engineered seafood and joined the Campaign for GE-Free Seafood. Stores included in the campaign were Whole Foods, Target, Trader Joe's, Aldi, Hy-Vee, Marsh, and Giant Eagle.

A case in federal court in San Francisco has raised a question about "all-natural" claims on Mission tortilla chips. Judge Yvonne Gonzalez Rogers put the case on hold for at least six months to give the FDA time to determine if

GMOs belong in the "all-natural" category.[22] The judge said there is a "gaping hole in the current regulatory landscape for 'natural' claims and GMOs."

"It should really be a no brainer that GMO crops cause significant damage to human health," according to Dr. Belin Poletto Mezzomo, an expert on the toxins and Bacillus thuringiensis (Bt) studies.[23] Animal testing has already proven the dangers of GMO consumption. This study unfortunately required the use of Swiss albino mice if Bt was to be properly examined. "At the same time, most of us know that the existence of GMOs is completely unnecessary," he added.[24]

The Collective Evolution website published a study in May 2013 stating that "Bacillus thuringiensis (Bt) toxins found in Monsanto crops are harmful to mammalian blood by damaging red blood cells and more."[25] Red blood cells (RBCs) are responsible for delivering oxygen to the body tissues through blood flow.[26]

Dr. Mezzomo and scientists at the University of Brasilia's Department of Genetics and Morphology and the Institute of Biological Sciences conducted the study. They evaluated hematotoxicity in Swiss albino mice to determine if red blood cells were being destroyed. Levels ranged from 27 mg to 270 mg for seven days, after which it was "remarkably evident that the Cry [Crystal] toxins were hemotoxic," or were disrupting blood clotting and destroying blood cells even at low doses around 27 mg. "Hemotoxins can cause organ degeneration and tissue damage," according to the report.[27] Cry toxins are a diverse group of proteins with activity against insects.

In this study it was noted that the numbers of RBCs, as well as their size, were significantly reduced, and so were the levels of hemoglobin for oxygen to attach to. Every factor regarding RBCs indicated some level of damage for all levels of toxin administered and across all Cry proteins. The tests clearly demonstrated that Cry proteins resulting from the Bt toxin were cytotoxic (quality of being toxic to cells) to bone marrow cells. Studies continually show that these proteins kill blood cells by targeting the cell membranes of RBCs.

Another study on Bt toxins found in Monsanto crops, conducted at the University of Western Ontario, produced similar results.[28] Genetics professor emeritus Joe Cummins concluded that sufficient evidence exists that "the Bt toxin will impact directly on human health through damaging the ileum, which is the final section of the small intestine that is responsible for the absorption of vitamin B12."

Ken Roseboro, publisher of the *Organic & Non-GMO Report and Sourcebook*, believes there is an unstoppable tide building in favor of mandatory GMO labeling of foods. In an August 2013 article in *Food-Navigator USA*, Roseboro says consumer interest is building everyday.[29] "Now there are 30 or 40 non GMO groups out there and a lot of them started in just the last two years. We've got Non GMO Vermont and Non GMO Mississippi."

But some members of Congress have in mind a dam to block the seemingly unstoppable tide favoring GMO labeling. The Safe and Accurate Food Labeling Act, as it has been coined, was introduced in early April 2014 by U.S. Representative Mike Pompeo (R-KS). If passed, the bill would prohibit mandatory labeling of GMO foods. Pompeo takes the issue a step further by shutting down the idea of the public getting involved through a public initiative on the state level. Pompeo's proposed law will obviously be fully supported by the Grocery Manufacturers Association.

The CSPI reminds us that the FDA is the agency assigned the responsibility for ensuring that all the foods we eat are safe.[30]

> However, the FDA does not have the legal authority to formally approve GE crops before they are commercialized. The FDA regulates GE food and feed crops through a voluntary notification process rather than by a mandatory pre-market approval process. In that voluntary process, the developer of a GE crop submits to the FDA a summary of data that shows that the GE crop is substantially equivalent to its traditionally bred counterpart and does not pose any novel health risk. The FDA reviews the submitted data and alerts the developer to any concerns it has about the developer's food safety assessment.[31]

There are enough questions raised about the safety of GMOs when it comes to the food we eat that the government must step up its enforcement. The CSPI has some of the most logical advice to our lawmakers. "Before any GE crop is turned into food, the FDA should have to formally approve that the crop is safe for human and animal consumption. Congress needs to amend the Federal Food, Drug, and Cosmetic Act to require a mandatory pre-market approval process that is open to public participation and review."[32]

Twenty-six states have GE labeling bills pending. Two states, Connecticut and Maine, passed bills in 2013 requiring labeling of foods that have been genetically modified. The previous year, California's GE labeling bill, known as Proposition 37, was defeated after big food manufacturing giants dumped millions of dollars into a smear campaign to mislead voters. Out-of-state food and chemical companies spent $45 million in California and $22 million in Washington State for the "No" campaigns.[33] The Washington State effort toward labeling of GE foods was narrowly defeated in November 2013.

The Center for Food Safety (CFS) reports, "The United States is one of the only developed countries in the world that doesn't require labeling" of genetically engineered foods.[34] An ABC News survey found 93 percent of the American public wanting the federal government to require mandatory labeling of GE foods.

President Obama made campaign promises to support a law requiring labeling of genetically modified foods.[35] In 2011, the CFS petitioned the

FDA urging labeling and even provided a detailed blueprint to make it an easy act on the issue.[36] CFS has received no reply from the FDA.

Ninety percent of Americans believe that GMOs are unsafe, 93 percent of Americans favor stringent federal GMO labeling regulations, and 57 percent say they would be less likely to buy products labeled as genetically modified, *Forbes* reported in January 2014.[37] The United States is one of the only developed countries in the world that doesn't require labeling on GMO foods.

Why such strong sentiment despite undeniable scientific findings to the contrary? According to *Forbes*, it is because 59 percent of Americans now follow nutritional advice they access on the Internet; the Internet is decidedly anti-GMO.[38]

An effort is well under way by the Grocery Manufacturers Association (GMA) to label GMO foods as "natural."[39] The Environmental Working Group quickly opposed the measure saying that "natural" means the product is "free of genetically engineered ingredients."[40] Other opponents say GMA is only trying to confuse the issue. The European Network of Scientists for Social and Environmental Responsibility (ENSSER) jumped into the middle of the issue pointing out that there is no scientific consensus on the safety of GMOs.[41]

More than 60 countries in the world label foods containing GMOs. But in Europe, when food manufacturers and outlets started labeling, "nobody would use the food—something companies fear as labeling initiatives go forward in the U.S.," according to CBS News medical consultant Dr. David Agus.[42]

While Congress has much work ahead on this issue, consumers are making a big difference with protests and calls for labeling of GMO products. The squeaky wheel gets the oil, and politicians and the giants of the food industry are tuned in. Whole Foods Market agreed in early 2014 to stop selling the Greek yogurt Chobani, which uses milk from cows fed with GMO animal feed.[43] Frito-Lay is sourcing non-GM ingredients, as is Gerber baby food. General Mills produces non-GMO Cheerios, made primarily with oats, for which there are no GMO varieties.[44] Chipotle Mexican Grill, Inc., switched in 2012 to non-GMO ingredients in its chain of 1,550 restaurants.[45] And the list grows.

Chapter Fifteen

Generally Recognized as Safe

There's a strange odor coming off of the FDA's GRAS. "Generally recognized as safe" (GRAS) designates additives in food that have not gone through premarket review and receive the FDA's stamp of approval, which is not required by law. Instead they are "generally recognized, among qualified experts, as having been adequately shown as safe."[1] Apparently we must assume "qualified experts" are, indeed, just that. Not only are they supposed to be qualified, they should be experts in this field and we have to assume they have no conflict of interest with the manufacturer of the additive. Now, if the additive was used in the food, it is given a GRAS approval based on "experience of common use in food including a substantial history of consumption for food use by a significant number of consumers." In other words, "We've used it all these years, so it should be considered safe." The FDA does not have to inspect or test the additive.[2] This is typical bureaucratic Washington at its best.

Scientists identified 275 chemicals from 56 companies that appear to be marketed for use in food, based on undisclosed GRAS safety determinations, according to Tom Neltner, JD, and Maricel Maffini, PhD, at the Natural Resources Defense Council.[3] "This is likely the tip of the iceberg. We previously published in an industry journal an estimate that there have been 1,000 such secret GRAS determinations. For each chemical we identified in this study, we did not find evidence that FDA had cleared them," they said.[4]

A study published in *JAMA* (*Journal of the American Medical Association*) found that employees of food manufacturers, people who had a vested interest in the outcome of the assessments, are many times the ones to pronounce an additive safe, even when the product has not undergone any testing and the risks to humans are simply unknown.[5] The analysis found that all of the 451 notifications voluntarily submitted to the FDA during that time were made by people who had relationships with manufacturers of food additives, which include salt, trans fats, and artificial flavors and sweeteners.[6] Pew found no independent reviews in GRAS determinations, which raised serious questions about the truthfulness, accuracy, and integrity of the GRAS process.[7] The most important question is this: Is the safety of the food ensured, especially when it comes to those food items in which the manufacturer fails to notify the FDA of the results?

We can draw our own conclusions based on the results: 22.4 percent of the GRAS assessments in question were conducted by an employee of the manufacturer of the ingredient being scrutinized, 13.3 percent were conducted by an employee of a consultancy selected by the manufacturer, and 64.3 percent were conducted by an expert panel selected by a consultancy or the ingredient manufacturer.[8]

Simply put, the FDA often lets the manufacturer decide if an additive is safe. (Oops, there I go again pointing to another case of our government giving preferential treatment to big business while ignoring the safety of the consumers.)

In 1958 Congress passed a law requiring companies adding a substance to food to provide some evidence of the safety of the food additive. But the law had no teeth. Manufacturers faced no requirement to provide absolute assurances that the substance was safe.

In 1997 it appeared the FDA was taking the bull by the horns and announced it was reinventing the regulations to streamline GRAS. Fifteen years later the new rules were still pending.

Food manufacturers have been able to slip a thousand additives into the U.S. food supply without any FDA record of the substances in those foods. For example, caffeine has been added to alcoholic beverages without informing the FDA.

The product known as Quorn™, which is basically a mycoprotein, serves many people as a meat-free form of high-quality protein and a good source of dietary fiber. The FDA categorizes mycoprotein as GRAS, but more than 1,500 adverse reactions have been reported to the Center for Science in the Public Interest, including severe abdominal pain, vomiting, diarrhea, and hives.[9] Several people have suffered breathing difficulties and even anaphylaxis (a life-threatening allergic reaction). Not surprisingly, a mycoprotein website lists a very low estimated risk of adverse reactions and says the most common side effect is just flatulence due to the fiber.[10]

Because GRAS notification is voluntary and companies are not required to identify nanomaterials in their GRAS substances, the FDA has no way of knowing the full extent to which engineered nanomaterials have entered the U.S. food supply as part of GRAS substances. In contrast to the FDA's approach, all food ingredients in Canada and the European Union that incorporate engineered nanomaterials must be submitted to federal regulators in those countries before they can be marketed. [11]

For years, CSPI has been urging the FDA to revoke Quorn™'s GRAS status, or at least to require warning labels.

The watchdog of all U.S. government agencies, the General Accountability Office (GAO), answers only to Congress. [12] Here's what GAO investigators found during their latest review of the FDA's GRAS program:

> The FDA's oversight process does not help ensure the safety of all new GRAS determinations. The FDA only reviews those GRAS determinations that companies submit to the agency's voluntary notification program—the agency generally does not have information about other GRAS determinations companies have made because companies are not required to inform the FDA of them. Furthermore, the FDA has not taken certain steps that could help ensure the safety of GRAS determinations, particularly those about which the agency has not been notified. [13]

GRAS is sometimes used as a loophole to get another food additive to the public without proceeding through the pages of government documents and the red tape and delay of having the product tested in a lab. The Natural Resources Defense Council argues the same point: "That FDA's inability to regulate ingredients that are GRAS, and therefore can be added to food products without approval, is an oversight loophole for unsafe chemicals in food that deserve more scrutiny." NRDC goes on to warn that federal protections to keep potentially unsafe chemicals out of food products are "woefully inadequate and may be putting the health of Americans at risk." [14]

The FDA has less assurance that companies have conducted and documented their determinations appropriately. Finally, without reconsidering and updating the 1997 proposed rule, the FDA may be falling short of fulfilling its food safety responsibilities.

One of the GAO's recommendations was for the FDA to develop a strategy to minimize the potential for conflicts of interest in companies' GRAS determinations, including taking steps such as issuing guidance for companies with conflicts of interests. [15]

It's impossible to compare the U.S. GRAS concept with other countries other than this one point. No other developed country in the world has a system like GRAS to provide oversight of food ingredients.

The FDA is not systematically ensuring the continued safety of current GRAS substances. Up until now, the FDA has largely not responded to concerns about GRAS substances, such as salt and the trans fats in partially hydrogenated vegetable oils, that individuals and consumer groups have raised through 11 citizen petitions submitted to the agency between 2004 and 2008. In fact, the FDA has decided on the validity of these concerns in only one of 11 cases. In addition, the FDA does not know to what extent, or even whether, companies track evolving scientific information about their GRAS substances.

But in late 2013, the FDA announced it would consider revoking the GRAS status of partially hydrogenated oils, known as PHOs.[16] This is a major step toward eradicating trans fats from the U.S. food supply.

Some of the products that would be affected include refrigerated biscuits, cinnamon rolls and frostings, cakes and frozen pies, snack foods, and frozen pizzas. Trans fats result when hydrogen is added to vegetable oil producing artificially hydrogenated oil that clogs arteries. Trans fats also raise bad cholesterol and lower good cholesterol.

The FDA began the lengthy process of obtaining public comments in an effort to develop a clearer picture of a time frame for a phase-out of the artificial trans fats in foods. Realistically, observing the past history of such detailed studies conducted by federal agencies, I would say we're looking at years before any ban is put into law. But the FDA says the ban can prevent as many as 7,000 deaths and 20,000 heart attacks a year.[17]

For now, the FDA urges consumers to check the Nutrition Facts panel on most foods where any trans fat content in the product must be included. But beware of a loophole in the law. The FDA has made it easy for food manufacturers to add some trans fat to foods without including it on the panel. Any food with trans fat additives under 0.5 grams per serving can be labeled "0 grams trans fats."[18] Yes, that is very misleading, but the FDA does not shy away from giving big food manufacturers the benefit of the doubt in many gray areas of food safety.

In a November 2013 "Food for Thought" article published in the *Huffington Post*, Gyorgy Scrinis, lecturer in food and nutrition politics at the University of Melbourne, Australia, points out some interesting facts about what he believes the FDA will not do concerning a proposed ban on trans fats.[19] "Industrial trans-fats themselves are in fact not being 'banned', and nor are there any limits to be placed on the trans-fats content of foods," Scrinis writes in his blog. "Nor are other minor sources of trans-fats being banned or regulated. At the same time few questions are being asked as to the safety and health implications of the processing techniques and ingredients that will replace trans-fats and partially hydrogenated vegetable (oil)," he adds.

Scrinis reminds us that the FDA has finally acknowledged that it is not in fact placing any bans or limits on trans fat levels in foods per se.

The FDA proposal will also face a steady barrage of questions regarding potential consequences regarding details of the agency's plan. Eric Decker, professor and department head at the University of Massachusetts' Department of Food Science, poses a couple of those expected questions.[20] "This proposed rule is not without consequences to many individuals so it is critical that this decision is made carefully." First, Decker questions the scientific data that the FDA is using to back up this proposed rule. Additionally,

Decker would like to know what substitute additive food manufacturers will come up with to replace trans fats when they are removed from the GRAS classification.

"Certain foods require solid fats for function (e.g., baked goods) so partially hydrogenated oil will have to be replaced with another solid fat such as palm oil. However, the health consequences of replacing partially hydrogenated oil with tropical oils in diets that already have low levels of trans fatty acids is unknown," Decker wrote.[21] (These comments were published in the November 13, 2013, issue of *The Weekly*, a blog of IFT, the Institute of Food Technologists.[22] For more than 70 years, IFT has been creating a dynamic global forum where members from more than 100 countries can share, learn, and grow.)

Many fast food chains, including McDonald's, stopped using trans fats when the FDA first required labeling in 2006.[23] Meanwhile, as the FDA meticulously wades through its bureaucratic process, heavy laden with red tape, many consumers will continue to eat bags of microwave popcorn, sticks of margarine, donuts by the dozen, and gallons of chocolate drink mixes.

Chapter Sixteen

BPA—Bisphenol A

When two giant food corporations discontinue using the dangerous containers that provide food for millions of their consumers, it's big. It's enormous. Bisphenol A (BPA), a chemical in the linings of many food cans and found in many plastic containers, contributes to brain development abnormalities, behavioral changes, cardiovascular disease, and cancer. The chemical enters food when it leaches from the lining of the containers.

Campbell's and H.J. Heinz companies no longer allow BPA in their packaging.[1] The move by these two major players in the food industry hopefully will pave the way to make BPA nonexistent in food packaging in the near future. Additionally, Greiner Packaging planned to cease using BPA in 2014.[2] "We will be the first leading company in our industry changing completely over to BPA-free materials in food packaging," says Willi Eibner, CEO of Greiner Packaging International. "The changeover mainly affects 5-gallon water bottles that were still being produced from polycarbonate." It's a major start toward protecting the lives of millions of the newly born and others.

BPA is also used in a multitude of other manufactured items, including compact disks, rugged sporting goods, water bottles, medical devices, and baby formulas.[3]

In April 2013 BPA was officially designated as a reproductive hazard in California.[4] Proponents of an outright ban look to California for the next step, requiring warning labels on products containing BPA. That could be years away, but it is a boost toward wiping out the potentially deadly results of BPA.

BPA, an industrial compound whose chemical composition is $C_{15}H_{16}O_2C_{15,}$ uses phenol and acetone as the building blocks for structural parts, impact resistant glazing, household appliance parts, electrical and electronic devices, and automotive applications.[5] Here's the most unsettling fact about it: despite government concerns, BPA received FDA approval just two weeks after results of a major study were announced stating that, even in tiny doses, hormone-disrupting chemicals like BPA are unsafe.[6]

Scientists at the Center for Progressive Reform agree that BPA poses a hazard even at low doses. Food safety authorities say levels of BPA should be eliminated to protect young children and pregnant women.[7] Pending legislation in a dozen states could soon ban BPA.

Interestingly, the FDA, the approving federal agency, admits on its own web pages that "the government, scientists and doctors need more research to better understand the potential human health effects of exposure to BPA, especially when it comes to the impact of BPA exposure on young children."[8] The FDA even gives pointers to help parents "minimize your infant's exposure to BPA." The agency published "What You Can Do to Minimize Your Infant's Exposure to BPA."

Just a suggestion here: Why not eliminate the problem altogether? "Minimizing" exposure may not be enough. You may be surprised to learn that our government suggests that one way mothers can avoid BPA is for them to breastfeed for 12 months. Why does the FDA take the easy way out by suggesting a temporary easing of the problem and at the expense of the mother, rather than take the obvious step and ban the chemical?

The FDA's own warnings should be enough information to put BPA on hold. The National Toxicology Program (NTP) says one reason people may be concerned about BPA is because human exposure to BPA is widespread.[9] Obviously acknowledging the dangers of BPA, another recommendation from the FDA is to discard a scratched baby bottle or feeding cups because they "may release small amounts of the chemical."[10] This takes the issue to another level in warnings in a report. Be careful how you heat up your child's breast milk or formula. Studies have found there is a very small amount of BPA in plastics and other packaging materials that can transfer to food and liquids, especially when heated. Additional traces of BPA levels are transferred when hot or boiling liquids or foods come in contact with packaging made of BPA.

Do not put boiling or very hot water, infant formula, or other liquids into BPA-containing bottles containers while preparing them for your child.

The European Union in July 2012 banned BPA only in baby bottles and sippy cups. The French government continues to work on a prohibition of BPA in all packaging; Sweden placed a ban on BPA in food packaging designed to be used by children under the age of three, similar to a ban in Denmark. The government of Denmark expressed its concerns about the safety of BPA in food contact areas by pointing to fears that the chemical could inhibit brain development and learning capacity. The government will continue the ban until new studies "document that low doses of Bisphenol A do not have an impact on development of the nervous system or on the behavior of rats" in lab tests. [11]

The human exposure to BPA can be found almost everywhere, increasing concerns where BPA is used. [12] The 2003–2004 National Health and Nutrition Examination Survey (NHANES), conducted by the Centers for Disease Control and Prevention, found detectable levels of BPA in 93 percent of 2,517 urine samples from Americans age six years and older. [13] Another reason for concern, especially for parents, may be that some laboratory animal studies report subtle developmental effects in fetuses and newborns exposed to low doses of BPA. The NTP has some concern for BPA's effects on the brain, behavior, and prostate gland in fetuses, infants, and children at current exposure levels.

A 2012 study linked BPA to changes in thyroid hormone levels in pregnant women and newborn boys. [14] Researchers at the University of California, Berkley, analyzed BPA levels in the urine samples of 335 women during the second half of pregnancy, and thyroid hormone levels in blood samples taken from the mothers during pregnancy and from the newborns within a few days of birth. The participants were part of the Center for the Health Assessment of Mothers and Children of Salinas (CHAMACOS) study led by Brenda Eskenazi, UC Berkeley professor of epidemiology and of maternal and child health.

The researchers found that for each doubling of BPA levels, there was an associated decrease of 0.13 micrograms per deciliter of total thyroxine (T4) in mothers during pregnancy, which suggests a hypothyroid effect—slowing the metabolism for people who develop this response. [15] For newborn boys, each doubling of BPA levels linked to a 9.9 percent decrease in thyroid stimulating hormone (TSH), indicating a hyperthyroid effect, according to the university's news center. No reason was given as to why an association with newborn girls was not established or ruled out. Animal studies may provide leads to an answer.

The Breast Cancer Fund, based in San Francisco, published six editions of its landmark report "State of the Evidence: The Connection between Breast Cancer and the Environment" until 2010. [16] The group studies possible relationships between breast cancer and exposure to chemicals and radiation. Among the Breast Cancer Fund's advisory board members is Dr. Susan E. Kutner, surgeon and chair of the Kaiser Permanente Northern California Breast Care Task Force. "Considerable data indicate exposure of humans to BPA is associated with increased risk for cardiovascular disease, miscarriages, decreased birth weight at term, breast and prostate cancer, reproductive and sexual dysfunctions, altered immune system activity, metabolic problems and diabetes in adults, and cognitive and behavioral development in young children," according to the Breast Cancer Fund. [17]

With regard to mammary development and increased risk for development of breast cancer, several studies using both rat and mouse models have demonstrated that even brief exposure to environmentally relevant doses of BPA during gestation or around the time of birth leads to changes in mammary tissue structure predictive of later development of tumors. Not only does early exposure to BPA lead to an increased risk for development of breast tumors, but exposure to BPA during chemotherapy treatment for breast cancer may make the treatment less effective, according to the group's paper on BPA.

In February 2013, ABC News conducted its own investigation into BPA and its effects on humans. Reporter Jim Avila found some amazing information about the chemical during an interview with Cheryl Rosenfeld, associate professor of biomedical sciences at the University of Missouri. "An expectant mother who has been exposed to BPA may jeopardize reproduction in many subsequent generations," she said.[18] "Chances are that moms are getting BPA without even knowing about it," she added.

Rosenfeld wanted to know if BPA could affect prenatal development in a mother's womb, because the chemical mimics the role of important sex hormones, specifically testosterone and estrogen. "It will bind to the same receptors that the natural hormone would bind to," she added. "But it is not regulated in a tight fashion like the natural hormones would be. So it kind of indiscriminately acts, and there's no ability to regulate it." It becomes a rogue hormone during the most critical phase in an organism's life, the development period prior to birth.

In September 2012, the prestigious *Journal of the American Medical Association* published a report titled "Association between Urinary Bisphenol A Concentration and Obesity Prevalence in Children and Adolescents," authored by Leonardo Trasande, MD, Teresa M. Attina, MD, and Jan Blustein, MD. The report stated, "In adults, elevated urinary BPA concentrations are associated with obesity and incident coronary artery disease. Childhood obesity may be caused by BPA exposure, however, all studies have not been completed."

In the 2003–2008 National Health and Nutrition Examination Survey's cross-sectional study of children and adolescents, urinary BPA concentration was significantly associated with obesity. The analysis involved a nationally representative subsample of 2,838 participants aged 6 through 19 years randomly selected for measurement of urinary BPA concentrations.

The start in the fall of 2010 of a new five-year study through an $8 million government-funded grant encouraged proponents of a total ban of BPAs for use in food contact areas. The investigation examines how substances used in food packaging affect the health and development of children.

The NTP conducted a review of lab studies in 2008 and expressed "concern for effects on the brain, behavior and prostate gland in fetuses, infants and children at current human exposures to Bisphenol A (BPA)." Program coordinators suggested even more investigations.

Another study on BPA levels in relation to obesity, conducted in Shanghai, suggests that BPS could be a new environmental obesogen, specifically a foreign chemical compound that disrupts normal development and balance of lipid metabolism, which can lead to obesity.[19] The study, published June 12, 2013, appeared in the Public Library of Science (PLOS-One), a peer-reviewed, nonprofit scientific journal. "The strongest evidence for the ability for environmental exposures to contribute to the development of diabetes comes from longitudinal studies," according to Diabetes and the Environment.[20] These are studies that take place over a period of time, where the exposure is measured before the disease develops.

The University of Illinois is conducting a study to determine the effects of plastics and chemicals on children's health.[21] "Our team has data from animal models showing that BPA and phthalates can have negative impacts on ovarian function and can exacerbate the effects of a high fat diet on body composition and metabolic status," said Dr. Susan Schantz, lead researcher of the University of Illinois project.

Consumers Union applauded the FDA's belated decision to ban BPA from infant formula but continues to work toward a ban of BPA in all food and beverage containers.[22] Consumers Union is the policy and action division of *Consumer Reports*, working with its million plus activists to pass consumer protection laws in states and in Congress. The consumer advocate group says, "Most consumers are currently exposed to BPA daily through common products like the linings of aluminum cans, water bottles, food storage containers, eating utensils, food cans, and other plastic containers. Exposure has been linked to health problems in animals and some human studies, including reproductive abnormalities and heightened risks of breast and prostate cancers, diabetes, and heart disease."

Congressman Edward Markey (D-MA) introduced the Ban Poisonous Additives Act of 2013 (BPA Act) that would "disallow the use of the BPA in empty and packed food containers and require periodic reexaminations of the safety of products currently deemed safe by the FDA."[23] Consumers Union wholeheartedly endorsed the measure, saying that in the past five years, some 34 states have introduced and 11 states have passed measures to regulate BPA in food and beverage containers and packaging.

The industry-supported International Food Information Council Foundation admits that BPA migrates out of cans into the food stored inside, but "at very low levels." Despite all the evidence from all the studies, the foundation continues to advise consumers that BPA in the lining of food packages is safe.

Chapter Seventeen

The Cottage Food Industry and Your Kitchen

Working at home takes on a whole new meaning when you replace your computer with mixing bowls and a hot oven. The cottage food industry flourishes in almost three dozen states where food prepared in the kitchen of the home or apartment is advertised and sold to the public from those homes or at farmers' markets. Cottage food laws have been enacted in 42 states. Those states forbidding the sale of food from your kitchen include the District of Columbia, Connecticut, Hawaii, Idaho, Kansas, Michigan, New Jersey, North Dakota, Oklahoma, and West Virginia.

Some states require a permit or license, but in most states, your kitchen won't be inspected by a licensing agency. One of the few restrictions in most states if you're using your kitchen at home for a business is the prohibition of any "potentially hazardous foods." This translates into "food that must be kept hot at 145 degrees or higher or cold foods that must be kept at 38 to 45 degrees or colder, depending on the product." However, in Michigan, pie crusts made with butter, a "potentially hazardous food," may be used in products such as pies that do not require refrigeration after baking.[1] The butter, prior to its use in making the crust, must be refrigerated to meet food safety standards.

Opposition to the Cottage Food Bill in Michigan came from within the state government.[2] The Michigan Department of Agriculture opposed the measure allowing food preparation sales from homes because "it posed an unwarranted hazard in a time of increasing food contamination incidents around the nation.[3] The Farm Bureau, siding with food producers, complained of unfair competition from work-at-home moms.[4] Proponents contended that the Cottage Food Bill represented a financial windfall for hundreds of Michigan families who have an inexpensive way to supplement their income.[5]

In Florida, no license, permit, or fees are required, but you are restricted to sales of only $15,000 a year.[6] You're not allowed to sell wholesale nor sell through the Internet or at grocery stores. Advertising is permitted and you may deliver your product to consumers.

In the cottage food industry, most state laws do not require inspections of homes for basic food safety requirements. For example, most other food sellers are visited by inspectors who check commissaries, food production lines, and other locations for hot water and soap for all kitchen employees, sanitizing stations for dirty pots and pans, cooking utensils at specific wash and rinse temperatures, cleaned and sanitized food contact surfaces, and the allowance of only authorized foods in the kitchen. Other major violations include the presence of rats, roaches, and flies and the storage of toxic materials near food preparation areas. The cottage food industry, however, never provides a registered food sanitarian to inspect for these critical requirements.

Caveat emptor.

Texas lawmakers closed a loophole in the proposed law regarding the all-important safety valve of packaging that has now grown to new heights in helping prevent intentional tampering of food products. Texas requires a label warning buyers that cottage-produced items "are not subject to rigorous health standards in food safety and packaging." Texas governor Rick Perry signed the law, which went into effect on September 1, 2013.

In California, Governor Jerry Brown signed the Homemade Food Act on September 21, 2012, and it became law on January 1, 2013. The governor came under fire from the California League of Cities, which complained that the law would single out a specific type of business for special treatment that other businesses do not receive.[7] In an August 31, 2012, letter to Brown from the League of California Cities, the legislative representative wrote: "This bill threatens to disturb neighbors that did not intend to locate their families next door to a business, deal with the traffic associated with a business, nor the smells that would permeate from a house. Local governments should be able to protect neighborhoods by regulating: hours of operation, the hours of on-site sales, inspections and advertising."[8]

A blog appearing on the Food Product Design website raises some important issues about novice cooks selling home-prepared foods to the public, even with some training. The author of the blog, Rachel Zemser, writing as the Intrepid Culinologist, took a food safety class on cottage food regulations in San Francisco County.

> I didn't realize how so completely in the dark consumers are about what makes a food safe. It doesn't help that the two-hour, mandatory a Cottage Food

Operator's food-safety course doesn't have to be taken before selling a home-made food, but within 90 days of selling a homemade food, and that it's based on restaurant operations, e.g., washing hands, keeping sanitation fluids away from food, temperature danger zones. But that still leaves CFO founders with no understanding of the rules behind creating these foods, including the three major contributing factors to an item's safety and shelf stability: water activity, pH and the thermal process. Cottage food entrepreneurs can sanitize their hands all day long, but if they sell beef jerky without checking the a_w [water activity], they could accidently kill someone. [9]

Opponents of the cottage food industry say that the development of shelf-stable foods should be left to the food scientists, or at least to those who have taken extensive food safety/food handling coursework. The cottage food industry is like a weapon of mass destruction that can potentially lead to disaster.

The Southeastern Retail Bakers Association complains that bakers have a difficult time selling cakes at $25 each because of their costs when the competition, cottage food operators, those who make and sell baked goods from their homes operators, sell the same cake at $10 and still make a healthy profit.

Utah's tough food law leaves the door open for home inspections of cottage food operators' kitchens. There should be "inspections of the home kitchen and re-inspections as the state deems necessary," according to the law. Alabama, Kentucky, Tennessee, New Jersey, and New York also have major restrictions on cottage food operations.

Determining whether food safety practices are followed in the kitchen of a private home is virtually impossible. In most states there are no inspections, much less surprise inspections to check for hot water, soap, towels and proper hand washing. There are no employees to snitch on the boss or other workers who fail to wash their hands. So who's to know?

There are four steps to food safety that home chefs should follow: [10]

1. CLEAN

Wash hands and surfaces often. Bacteria can spread throughout the kitchen and get onto hands, cutting boards, utensils, countertops, and food. To ensure that your hands and surfaces are clean, be sure to:

- Wash your hands with warm water and soap for at least 20 seconds before and after handling food and after using the bathroom, changing diapers, and handling pets.
- Wash your cutting boards, dishes, utensils, and countertops with hot soapy water after preparing each food item and before you go on to the next food.

- Consider using paper towels to clean up kitchen surfaces. If you use cloth towels, wash them often in the hot cycle of your washing machine.
- Rinse fresh fruits and vegetables, including those with skins and rinds that are not eaten, under running tap water.
- Rub firm-skin fruits and vegetables under running tap water or scrub with a clean vegetable brush while rinsing with running tap water.
- With canned goods, remember to clean lids before opening.

2. SEPARATE

Separate raw meats from other foods. Cross-contamination can occur when bacteria are spread from one food product to another. This is especially common when handling raw meat, poultry, seafood, and eggs. The key is to keep these foods—and their juices—away from ready-to-eat foods.

To prevent cross-contamination, remember to:

- Separate raw meat, poultry, seafood, and eggs from other foods in your grocery shopping cart, grocery bags, and your refrigerator.
- Use one cutting board for fresh produce and a separate one for raw meat, poultry, and seafood.
- Never place cooked food on a plate that previously held raw meat, poultry, seafood, or eggs.
- Don't reuse marinades used on raw foods unless you bring them to a boil first.

3. COOK

Cook to the right temperatures. Food is safely cooked when it reaches a high enough internal temperature to kill the harmful bacteria that cause illness. Refer to the Safe Cooking Temperatures Chart for the proper internal temperatures.[11]

To ensure that your foods are cooked safely, always:

- Use a food thermometer to measure the internal temperature of cooked foods. Check the internal temperature in several places to make sure that the meat, poultry, seafood, and eggs or dishes containing eggs are cooked to safe minimum internal temperatures as shown in the Safe Cooking Temperatures Chart.
- Cook ground meat or ground poultry until it reaches a safe internal temperature. Color is not a reliable indicator of doneness.
- Cook eggs until the yolk and white are firm. Only use recipes in which eggs are cooked or heated thoroughly.
- When cooking in a microwave oven, cover food, stir, and rotate for even cooking. If there is no turntable, rotate the dish by hand once or twice

during cooking. Always allow standing time, which completes the cooking, before checking the internal temperature with a food thermometer. Food is done when it reaches the safe minimum internal temperature.

- Bring sauces, soups, and gravies to a boil when reheating.

4. CHILL

Refrigerate foods promptly, because cold temperatures slow the growth of harmful bacteria. Do not over-stuff the refrigerator. Cold air must circulate to help keep food safe. Keeping a constant refrigerator temperature of 40°F or below is one of the most effective ways to reduce the risk of foodborne illness. Use an appliance thermometer to be sure the temperature is consistently 40°F or below and the freezer temperature is 0°F or below.

To chill foods properly:

- Refrigerate or freeze meat, poultry, eggs, seafood, and other perishables within two hours of cooking or purchasing. Refrigerate within one hour if the temperature outside is above 90°F.
- Never thaw food at room temperature, such as on the countertop. Food must be kept at a safe temperature during thawing. There are three safe ways to defrost food: in the refrigerator, in cold water, and in the microwave. Food thawed in cold water or in the microwave should be cooked immediately.
- Always put marinating food in the refrigerator.
- Divide large amounts of leftovers into shallow containers for quicker cooling in the refrigerator.
- Use or discard refrigerated food on a regular basis.

Foodborne illness can strike anyone. However, some people are at higher risk than others. These include pregnant women, young children, older adults, and people with weakened immune systems. If you—or someone you care for—are in one of these at-risk groups, it's important to pay extra attention to handling food safely.

I'll leave this subject with a true story about flies. It comes from a prize-winning poster from the Health Education Council describing what happens when a fly lands on your food:

> Flies can't eat solid food, so to soften it up they vomit on it. Then they stamp on the vomit until it's a liquid, usually stamping in a few germs for good measure. Then when it's good and runny, they suck it all back again, probably dropping some excrement at the same time. And then when they've finished eating, it's your turn. [12]

Chapter Eighteen

Restaurant Food

Ah, I finally got around to the subject close to your heart and stomach. You love to eat out. No grocery stores. No produce to scrub. No cooking, defrosting, or dishes to do. So here you are at the alternative to all that work at home, be it at a five-star restaurant or the drive-through lane at a fast-food restaurant. You have decided to put your food safety in the hands of others. You're not thinking about the pesticides on the fields of wheat, the cattle pens and slaughterhouses, or polluted waters. You're not wondering if the FDA was on hand when your Mediterranean salad was bagged, if that chicken was really inspected, and when the meat slicer back at the deli was last cleaned. But should you be thinking about these things?

Many of us do not have time to cook. So, often Americans end up eating a good portion of their meals in restaurants, where they are more likely than at home to be hit with a foodborne illness, which could lead to hospitalization and even death.[1]

I spent twenty years as an investigative reporter at two ABC News affiliate stations, KAKE-TV in Wichita and WFAA-TV, Dallas. Much of my time at those two television stations involved producing, writing, and reporting on restaurant inspections and investigating what those violations on paper really looked like up close. I always accompanied a registered food sanitarian, usually with the city or state health department, when we visited any food service establishment. We walked through kitchens of hospitals, nursing homes, schools, country clubs, airline food commissaries, and fast-food and five-star restaurants. Street vendors' food items from Dallas to New York, food manufacturing plants, and slaughterhouses were featured on our reports. Food safety research was documented at the University of California-Riverside and in Arizona and Illinois. We found rats, roaches, decaying food on metal shelves above uncovered salads, chicken sitting out at room temperature, flies swarming in and out of restrooms with doors ajar, and practically no hand washing at most of the restaurants (why would employees want to wash their hands in a dirty sink with no soap or towels? Not too conducive to personal hygiene and food safety).

Every type of retail location that sold food was included in the reports. We expanded the depth of our food investigations with trips to Los Angeles, Phoenix, Albuquerque, Chicago, and New York to document first hand how tough food inspectors operated in other cities. And yes, they possess the authority and use it with the force of City Hall backing them in the corner deli, the expensive French restaurant, and with street vendors. Probably the worst sight for a restaurant patron to set eyes upon would be the resilient and germ-laden German cockroach scampering across the salad bar or on your table.[2]

I ran across some interesting research in the basement of a building at the University of California at Riverside. Entemologist Don Reierson opened the lid to a large barrel of cockroaches, feasting and running about a wooden centerpiece inside.[3]

Professor Reierson developed a method to stop the rapid reproduction of the most resilient pest on earth, the common German cockroach, which enthusiastically patrols most restaurants producing those odorous secretions on our food. Reierson's study discovered a lethal yeast growing inside the German roach. "When extracted and fed to other roaches, the yeast brings almost instant death to the roaches," Reierson told me as he dug into a container of tens of thousands of roaches used in the study.

"The yeast has probably been around for a long while and no one has recognized its presence," Reierson said. During a typical commercial spraying of a restaurant using industry chemicals, at least 10 percent of the roach population survives. "The survivors are capable of withstanding high levels of insecticides and often their offsprings are capable of withstanding even higher levels."

Professor Reierson retired in 2010 without locating an interested company that would take the project to a commercial venture. Michael Rust, who was part of the research in the 1980s, now holds the position of distinguished professor of entomology at the university. In April 2014 he told me, "With the later discovery of hydramethylnon as a cockroach bait, any interest in a biological alternative quickly disappeared."[4] Professor Rust also suggested, "As so often happens in urban pest management research, the appearance of a successful control strategy will actually impede future research until that strategy begins to fail."

Once again that tough little German cockroach wins.

My television reports on the many phases of our food safety problems were eye-opening for the public. For me, it was a welcome challenge to present the reports on two newscasts a night displaying our tours of grease-laden kitchens where employees used can openers crusted with decaying food and unprotected food stored uncovered under toxic chemicals, to name a couple of the violations. But it's a different picture out there where the diners have gathered in the exquisitely appointed dining rooms with glistening silverware and crystal adorning freshly pressed white tablecloths. Little do they know, unfortunately, what lurks behind those kitchen doors.

It had been well over two years since the last inspection at some restaurants. The reaction of management at these food service establishments brought varied results, some of them pretty humorous. Dallas Morning News television critic Ed Bark said in one of his 1983 columns, "Duncan Does Tasteful Job with Restaurant Series," "Rodents on the taffy pull machine sounds funny on the face of it, but Duncan says it as though he were reading a robbery suspect his rights."[5]

I observed Peking ducks hanging in the window of a restaurant specializing in Chinese food and asked the manager if he thought the ducks should be refrigerated. "That's your problem," he replied. I imagine our viewers wondered why he thought the problem was mine and after a couple of decades, I'm still puzzled. Minutes later, we videoed an employee removing the ducks from hazardously hanging in the window of the restaurant.

I spoke with the manager of the kitchen in a large nursing home in Dallas where flies had virtually taken over food preparation areas and dining room tables. With our camera rolling I asked, "Why so many flies?" Without hesitation he came back, "It's the back door that doesn't close tight enough to keep them out." I asked, "Has anyone thought about having the door repaired, so it closes properly?" The kitchen manager said he had turned in a work order to maintenance.

The series brought out some startling facts regarding our food chain. "Millions of people are getting sick each year from contamination in intestinal contents during the animal slaughtering process," according to Dr. Ed Manning, a former National Association of Federal Veterinarians spokesman. "No requirement exists in the regulations to determine any level of disease bacteria that may be in raw meats or poultry," he told me.[6]

I discovered a disturbing fact in that local food inspectors in cities across the country did not have one standard, uniform set of rules and laws to guide them through the inspection process. The Center for Science in the Public Interest (CSPI) had suggested the rules as far back as 1996, then later produced and circulated one of the most important and comprehensive reports on food inspections with issues that are current and even more needed today than when they were first published.[7] Here are the key points in the study:

> Hidden dangers lurk in restaurant food, dangers that can cause acute illness and sudden death. Harmful bacteria, viruses and parasites in ready-to-eat restaurant food cause several thousand deaths and millions of illnesses each year.

Government data in 2014 show that consumers are twice as likely to report getting sick from a food poisoning outbreak caused by restaurant food than from food prepared at home. And with more consumers eating away from home than ever before, the numbers of illnesses and deaths are likely to rise, unless restaurants and the state, city, and county agencies that regulate them, improve the systems that are designed to best ensure food safety.

The CSPI states that most poisonings from food stored and prepared in restaurants can be simply and easily prevented.[8] In a nutshell, check cooking and refrigeration temperatures, assure proper food handling including correct hand washing, and avoid possible cross-contaminations such as the dangerous combination of salads and raw chickens prepared on the same cutting board.

In a survey of 45 state and local government agencies that conduct inspections of restaurants, CSPI found that a large majority of agencies are not following FDA's national standards for restaurants (the "Food Code").[9] Agencies in Concord, New Hammpshire, and the state of Rhode Island were the best that CSPI surveyed.

Only 13 percent of the agencies surveyed enforce the FDA's Food Code recommended cooking temperatures for pork, eggs, fish, and poultry, and only 64 percent require hamburgers to be cooked to 155°F, the temperature necessary for E. coli O157:H7 to be destroyed in 15 seconds.[10] Only 11 percent of the agencies require refrigeration of food at the temperature recommended by FDA. Only 20 percent follow Food Code temperature recommendations for cooling cooked food. Less than half of the agencies inspect restaurants twice a year. Only 16 percent require consumer warnings for raw food, like shellfish, and undercooked food, like rare hamburgers.[11]

Even where states and localities are using the most current version of the FDA Food Code, inspectors complain that their work is compromised by lack of funding and inadequate inspection tools.[12] Ultimately, restaurants themselves will have to provide greater assurance to both their customers and the government regulators that they are serving the safest possible meals.

The nationwide publicity that followed the outbreak of a deadly strain of E. coli bacteria traced to fast-food hamburgers in 1993, and publicity regarding the safety of certain products such as seafood, has provided the incentive for many restaurants to test new systems to improve their food safety performance.[13] Many ways and means exist that can improve the food safety in restaurants and other food establishments. As mentioned earlier in this book, the FDA utilizes what is known as hazard analysis and critical control points, or HACCP.[14] Preventive HACCP controls, coupled with laboratory testing, are being used in several national restaurant chains. Adoption of HACCP greatly improves the safety of food served in restaurants.

According to the Center for Science in the Public Interest, all state and local governments should incorporate the FDA Food Code's food safety standards into their laws governing inspection and should update their laws whenever the Food Code is updated.[15] State and local governments should mandate that restaurants utilize HACCP systems to improve the safety of the meals they serve. Local health authorities should assist restaurants in setting up and monitoring HACCP plans, and must verify that HACCP plans are working by conducting periodic laboratory testing of food and equipment samples taken from restaurants. Inspectors should have the proper equipment to measure cooking temperatures of food during inspections.

State and local governments should make restaurant food safety a higher budgetary priority and should ensure that local inspection agencies have sufficient funds to carry out their functions. They should work with restaurants and restaurant trade associations to develop food safety recognition programs for restaurants. Eligible restaurants should be those that have consistently maintained safe operations and that have instituted HACCP systems.

Even if not required to do so by law, all restaurants should establish HACCP plans to identify and control the risks of foodborne illness in their operations. Since harmful pathogens frequently contaminate the food supply, particularly seafood, meat, poultry, and eggs, HACCP plans should contain provisions for restaurants to monitor the quality of products they receive from suppliers, including the use of temperature monitoring devices during shipping and laboratory testing of suppliers' products. Restaurant HACCP plans should require that suppliers implement their own HACCP plans to ensure the safety of food from the farm through the processing and shipping stages.

To encourage the adoption of uniform standards, Congress should allocate money for increased restaurant inspections and enforcements to states that adopt the FDA Food Code's food safety and inspection standards. The money should not be taken from the existing budgets of federal food safety agencies. On both the state and federal levels, additional funding should be allocated for epidemiological studies of foodborne illness. The USDA and FDA should step up efforts to ensure that seafood, meat, poultry, and eggs are as free from harmful bacteria and other contaminants as possible.

Inspectors utilize a standard inspection form that has changed very little in the last 40 years.[16] The perfect score is 100; a passing score generally is considered 70. But much more goes into an inspection than just deducting points. The most serious violations receive four or five points off. One or two points are deducted for less serious problems like unclean floors, unclean non-food contact areas, and failure to post the most recent inspection. A restaurant could receive 10–15 minor violations and not receive a closing notice or citation.

Critical 4- and 5-point scores can close a restaurant with one or two violations. For example, if a restaurant's water heater fails to work properly, the restaurant would be closed since dishes, silverware, food contact surfaces, and hands cannot be properly washed and sanitized. Other serious violations include food received from an unapproved source; products maintained at improper temperatures (hot foods must be at 145°F or hotter and cold foods at 38–45° or colder, depending on the food); plumbing problems involving cross connections or backups; improper toilet facilities; presence of insects, rodents, or birds; and toxic items stored near food or food preparation areas. This is not a complete listing of violations.

In many cities, the public can access restaurant inspection information online. Consumers can learn much about a restaurant before they enter. Check around the back, at and near the dumpster. Are the sliding doors closed or the top closed? Any litter noticed around the dumpster? Does a grease trail lead out the back door to the dumpster? Inside, is the staff observing good hygiene practices (e.g., fingers away from the mouth and face)? Are the floors, tables and chairs, condiment containers on the table, and the menu clean? These signs often give the public an idea about how the kitchen looks.

I'm often asked how many times I was sued for invasion of privacy or libel producing food safety reports. The question usually came from an attorney or journalist. After airing more than 100 reports on food service facilities, I was sued one time. We had accompanied a state of Kansas food inspector to a Wichita restaurant where the owner gave us written permission to accompany the inspector and videotape the inspector's findings. The owner signed the written agreement. The inspector witnessed the signature. The restaurant owner, later that day, called our TV station owner, the late Martin Umansky, and stated he was withdrawing permission. We believed permission could not be withdrawn. We aired the segment. The restaurant owner sued. The jury deliberated less than an hour and ruled in our favor. There was no appeal.

Chapter Nineteen

Government's Report Card

For the first time since the 1930s, the U.S. government decided in 2008 to streamline our antiquated set of food safety laws.[1] The efforts immediately slowed to a crawl. Finally, the law known as the FDA Food Safety and Modernization Act was signed and passed by the president on January 4, 2011.[2] Congress failed to provide funding, and the first deadline for implementing the act was missed on January 1, 2012. Vital programs were slashed from the original law. Budgets face major cuts when and if funding ever occurs. Meanwhile, the White House claims that the "American food safety system is among the best in the world."[3] But there's plenty of strong disagreement. U.S. food safety is "definitely years behind Europe," according to Stefano Crea, food sector manager for the certification body Det Norske Veritas (DNV), one of three classification companies serving a wide spectrum of fields around the world.[4]

The problems are crystal clear; answers are shrouded in clouds of doubt. In 2009, President Obama formed the President's Food Safety Working Group, which quickly discovered and admitted in its key findings that several serious problems continue.[5] "Our system is hamstrung by outdated laws, insufficient resources, suboptimal management structures, and poor coordination across agencies and with States and localities. At least a dozen Federal agencies, implementing at least 30 different laws, have roles in overseeing the safety of the nation's food supply. This approach was not rationally designed," the group stated.[6] "Too often in the past, the food safety system has focused on reacting to problems rather than preventing harm in the first place." That was 2009.[7]

Our government wants to turn inspections over to the food producers, a system that has been tried and proven ineffective. The fox rules the roost when he guards the hen house. Federal food safety agencies must abandon

the idea of allowing producers of beef and poultry products to police themselves. The U.S. government would like to drastically cut inspectors from
production lines and slaughterhouses, leaving poultry plant employees to
conduct inspections.

One solution appears to be to simply bite the bullet and provide the FDA
and the USDA with more funding for inspectors to accomplish the goals of
their jobs. All of our food safety agencies need financial assistance. But
before more money is handed out to these agencies, shouldn't we first correct
all the mistakes coming out of Washington and make better use of the available funds? The U.S. General Accountability Office uses that reasoning often
in auditing the myriad of government agencies. Our government does almost
nothing to inspect the food imported from other countries[8] or correct a situa-
tion that is shocking and life-threatening: we eat food products from other
countries that have virtually no U.S. inspection. The FDA and the USDA
have been strictly mandated to provide a high level of food inspections and
enforcement, but the mandates are far from followed and enforcement is
nearly nonexistent.

When the FDA publicly admits that inspection of foods arriving from
about 200 countries at 300 different U.S. ports is "inadequate," and consumer
groups say it is more like "nonexistent," it is imperative that an immediate,
emergency change be made.[9] Once again the solution is clear. To adequately
protect the imported food we eat, which accounts for 13 percent of our diets,
we must have more inspectors at all 300 ports of entry conducting thorough
testing, making necessary seizures, and taking other actions required without
fear of bureaucratic interference.[10] As long as we continue to import 10
million pounds of food every year, we need comparable inspections to keep
pace.

Another problem centers on the lack of confidence and respect from the
consumer. The FDA, USDA, and CDC display blatant signs of nontranspa-
rency. The CDC often refuses to reveal the names of restaurant chains where
hundreds of diners have fallen ill from contaminated food.[11]

"There is a need for better food safety inspection all along the way.[12] We
have folks who have not been able to get Salmonella out of turkeys in the
U.S.," according to Jaydee Hanson, a senior policy analyst at the Center for
Food Safety. Bill Marler, a leading food safety advocate and food poisoning
attorney, says foodborne illness deaths and injuries always result from mistakes: "There is not one foodborne illness outbreak I've been involved with
in 20 years where it couldn't have been prevented had people been paying
attention," he said.[13]

The United States must implement ways to better cope with the rising
number of food poisonings that lead to economic losses, sicknesses, and
deaths. Squabbling lawmakers must set their sights on saving lives by pro-

viding funding for the food safety agencies every step of the way, from the crops in the fields to our dinner tables.

The Government Accountability Office, the independent agency with "watchdog authority" to dissect every other federal government entity, cited agency fragmentation in its 2012 report. The GAO report found 32 areas of costly duplication or overlap of programs.[14] Centrally coordinated oversight is needed to ensure the nine federal agencies effectively and efficiently implement the nation's fragmented policy to defend the food and agriculture systems against potential terrorist attacks, major disasters, and increasing numbers of sicknesses and deaths from foodborne illnesses.[15]

Support for the GAO report comes from the fact that the United States experienced the greatest increase in food recalls in the years 2008 through 2011. During the last quarter of 2011, the FDA reported 176 recalls by about 160 companies, an 80 percent increase over the previous quarter. Most of the food recalls were traced to undeclared allergens, Listeria, Salmonella, Botulinum, and E. coli, in that order.[16]

The Alliance for a Stronger FDA mandated itself virtually impossible goals: (1) To assure that the U.S. FDA has sufficient resources to protect consumers, and (2) to maintain public confidence and trust in the FDA.[17] The alliance pointed out that "the federal government gives the FDA about $8 per year for each American (an 'appropriation' of $2.457 billion for FY 2011). Nowhere else in the federal budget does so little money need to go so far. . . . The FDA allots just 10,000 employees to monitor food safety, review the safety and efficacy of medical products, assure the safe use of those medical products, and protect the American people, their pets, and their farm animals from poorly made, counterfeit, and illegal food, drugs, and cosmetics."[18]

The alliance, looking toward the next federal budget, says the FDA may do what it has done in the past: "hold back on hiring and issuing contracts to blunt the impact of potential cuts later in the fiscal year, which might come from either appropriations, cuts, or a new sequester."[19]

"Holding back" indicates that more of the same would be on the horizon for food inspections, recalls, and seizures of contaminated food at ports of entry and more foodborne illnesses, hospitalizations, and deaths. We need to push forward, not hold back.

Why must we go to court to try to convince our federal government to do its job? Two nonprofit public interest advocacy groups went to federal court in the northern district of California in 2012 seeking relief for repeated missed deadlines to implement the Food Safety Modernization Act.[20] The lawsuits charge the FDA with failing to meet several hundred deadlines that were included in the law but ignored by the food safety agency.[21]

The Center for Environmental Health and the Center for Food Safety contend that a new food safety law, mired in bureaucratic double-talk at the U.S. FDA and the Office of Management and Budget, could help prevent thousands of deaths caused by foodborne illnesses each year. New rules contained in the law would force food companies to take a more active role in locating causes for pathogen contaminations in the foods they produce. The law would require importers to assume the responsibilities involved for food safety. Fresh fruits and vegetables would fall under stricter rules.

The U.S. government's food safety efforts were last overhauled in 1940, so it is long overdue for not just a tune-up but perhaps a complete remake inside and out. When President Obama signed the Food Safety and Modernization Act in January 2011, he called it one of the hallmarks of his first administration. The signing ceremony brought hopes for safer foods, but those hopes were false, as the act has failed miserably. [22]

Looking ahead, there's more pie-in-the-sky and bureaucratic talk from the people in Washington who seem to think that this country is full of gullible people. The FDA's future hopes include an inspection every five years at each food service and food production facility with the first inspection taking place within several years of the signing of any new law. I've pointed out that the FDA often has its head in the sand, but this look toward the future has the agency's eyes glazed over or completely shut from reality.

The indisputable facts justify the cries for help from consumer groups, some of our lawmakers, and the millions of people who buy food they assume is safe. But all it takes is a quick look at the effects of our deplorable food safety programs to realize the truth is found in these statistics. They are not just numbers. They are people, numbering more than 48 million who are poisoned from foodborne pathogens, 127,839 hospitalized, and 3,037 dead from consuming contaminated food in 2011. [23] Those numbers are closely duplicated every year. It's difficult to explain why House Republicans cut the FDA's food safety budget claiming the U.S. food system is 99 percent safe. [24] It was a pathetic allegation, made without a thread of backup material, designed to give consumers false confidence in the safety of the food we eat. Obviously, we have many elected officials with their heads also in the sand.

That's how unsafe our food has become.

Epilogue

Sugar, the Legalized Recreational Drug

When writing about food safety, I would be remiss if I didn't include the hazards of sugar consumption. We're not talking about Salmonella or other foodborne illnesses. We're at the beginning of a long and historic campaign to regulate sugar like we regulate alcohol and tobacco.

Essentially, more and more scientists and physicians view sugar as a legalized recreational drug that's socially acceptable to consume, cautioning that just like other drugs, over time, it destroys a person's health, disrupts normal brain function, promotes heart disease, and directly causes diabetes and obesity.[1]

Dr. Robert Lustig is a pediatric endocrinologist and professor of clinical pediatrics at the University of California San Francisco School of Medicine: "It has nothing to do with the calories. It's a poison by itself," Dr. Lustig lectured as video cameras rolled for 90 minutes on that day in May 2009 at the university.[2] Since that time, the lecture, "Sugar: The Bitter Truth," has been posted on YouTube and gone viral, reaching more than four million viewings going into 2014. "It's one more nail in the coffin for the argument that fructose and glucose act the same, that calories count the same no matter where they come from," Lustig said. He added, "Sugar consumption, like alcohol, is a major contributor to fatty liver disease, which has been on the rise."[3]

According to a United Nations declaration, "Governments should consider controlling sweeteners with taxes and regulations just like they control alcohol and tobacco."[4] "Sugar feeds cancer cells, triggers weight gain, and promotes premature aging, draining and leaching the body of precious vitamins and minerals through the demand its digestion, detoxification and elim-

141

ination makes upon one's entire system," according to Dr. William Coda Martin in an article published in a Global Healing Center newsletter.[5] In the article, "Refined Sugar—The Sweetest Poison of All," Dr. Martin added, "Refined sugar is lethal when ingested by humans because it provides only that which nutritionists describe as empty or naked calories. It lacks the natural minerals, which are present in the sugar beet or cane."

In addition, so essential is balance to our bodies that we have many ways to provide against the sudden shock of a heavy intake of sugar.[6]

The argument that street drugs are outlawed because they're dangerous to a person's health falls flat on its face when you consider the damage sugar does to the human body. Sugar is much more dangerous than marijuana, for example, and yet marijuana is illegal to possess or consume in almost all states.

It's estimated that the average American consumes about 90 pounds of sugar a year. And when we put anything in our mouths with sugar in it, our pancreas is immediately stimulated to release insulin, according to CBS News medical correspondent Dr. Jennifer Ashton.[7] "It also stimulates the liver. And we know that a lot of sugar that's not burned immediately as fuel gets turned into fat. What happens is over an amount of time and years, and we don't know how much sugar and how much time, the pancreas can get worn out, it can lead to diabetes. There's new research that suggests that insulin really works as a growth factor to trigger, stimulate, feed, and nourish tumor cells, and therefore, is implicated in cancer," she says. Elevated sugar levels put you at high risks for lethal injuries and damage to your heart, kidneys, liver, brain, eyes, blood vessels, and basically every degenerative disease in the top 10 list of killers. As you see, the dangers of sugar are vast and enormous. Sugar causes a loss of tissue elasticity and function; the more sugar you eat the more elasticity and function you lose.

Mark Hyman, writing in the *New York Daily News*, says, "We now know—because it has been scientifically proven—that sugar is more powerfully addictive than alcohol, cocaine or even heroin."[8] And don't think a diet soda will take the place of sugar. "Take note: Artificial sweeteners may be more addictive than regular sugar," Dr. Hyman added.

Stephanie Johnson, editor-in-chief of Health Enews, quoting from the journal *PLoS*, cites a strong link between higher diabetes rates and sugar. "Many experts are calling the data a 'smoking-gun,' equivalent to the 1960s study that linked cigarettes to lung cancer."[9] In a statement, one of the lead authors of the study said, "You could not enact a real-world study that would be more conclusive than this one." Scientists involved in the study are hopeful their findings are the ammunition needed to prove sugar is toxic and hopefully get something done about it. Johnson is an award-winning journalist and director of public affairs for Advocate Health Care, one of the nation's top health systems.

It's difficult to always know at a glance how much sugar is in packaged food because it's often hidden under a different name. You don't have to be a food investigator to decipher the numbers on the Nutrition Facts panel of foods.[10] The line for sugars contains both the natural and added types as total grams of sugar. There are four calories in each gram, so if a product has 15 grams of sugar per serving, that's 60 calories just from the sugar alone, not counting the other ingredients.

To determine if a processed food contains added sugars, you need to look at the list of ingredients. But remember, sugar is still sugar no matter what name you give it. Several sugar products end in "-ose," such as sucrose.[11] And we have raw sugar, brown sugar, syrup, high fructose corn syrup, and others.

Natural News website adds to that list: "lactose (as in milk), maltose or malts (as in rice malt and honey), jam (contains concentrated juice, which is high in fruit sugar), maple syrup, corn syrup, palm sugar (traditionally used in macrobiotic cooking), and the very deceiving organic brown sugar, which is not all that different from white sugar. Even alcohol is a sugar. All of these sugars are problematic in many different ways."[12]

Nancy Appleton, PhD, clinical nutritionist, in her book *Lick the Sugar Habit*, lists 141 reasons why sugar is detrimental to your health. Here are just a few:

- Sugar feeds cancer.
- Sugar increases cholesterol.
- Sugar can weaken eyesight.
- Sugar can cause drowsiness and decreased activity in children.
- Sugar can interfere with the absorption of protein.
- Sugar causes food allergies.
- Sugar contributes to diabetes.
- Sugar can contribute to eczema in children.
- Sugar can cause cardiovascular disease.
- Sugar contributes to osteoporosis.
- Sugar can impair the structure of DNA.
- Sugar can cause hyperactivity, anxiety, difficulty concentrating, and crankiness in children.
- Sugar contributes to the reduction in defense against bacterial infection (infectious diseases).
- Sugar greatly assists the uncontrolled growth of Candida albicans (yeast infections).
- Sugar can decrease growth hormone (the key to staying youthful and lean).

Natural News gives us this encouraging reminder. "The wonderful thing is that we do not have to give up the sweetness of sugar in order to be healthy; we just need to replace it with better alternatives. While giving up sugar is very difficult, replacing it is now very easy. There are two natural, organic sugar alternatives that are sweet, easy to use and cook with—stevia and xylitol. They may sound like chemicals but they are completely natural and have been proven not only safe but also beneficial for our well-being."[13]

Despite all the facts I have listed, our government regards sugar as safe, and it is listed by the U.S. Department of Agriculture on the GRAS list. A reminder is in order here, in case you may have missed it in an earlier chapter: just because an additive or food is listed as GRAS doesn't mean it has been proven safe. Michael F. Jacobson, executive director of the Center for Science in the Public Interest, calls for a major change. In a press release he said that the CSPI names high fructose corn syrup, sucrose, and "other sugars" as unsafe at the levels consumed. It claims "to be GRAS, there must be a scientific consensus that the ingredient is safe at the levels consumed."[14]

Jacobson makes another point. "As currently formulated, Coke, Pepsi, and other sugar-based drinks are unsafe for regular human consumption. Like a slow-acting but ruthlessly efficient bioweapon, sugar drinks cause obesity, diabetes, and heart disease. The FDA should require the beverage industry to re-engineer their sugary products over several years, making them safer for people to consume, and less conducive to disease."

What does the Sugar Association say about all of these scientific facts about the dangers associated with sugar? The association issued a statement in 2011: "We consider it irresponsible when health professionals use their platforms to instill fear by using words like 'diabetes,' 'cancer,' and even 'death,' without so much as one disclaimer about the fact that the incomplete science being referenced is inconclusive at best. We are confident that the American people are perfectly capable of choosing what foods to eat without stark regulations and unreasonable bans imposed upon them."[15]

More evidence of the real dangers of consuming sugar is found in the February 2014 report by the CDC and published in *JAMA*. "Epidemiologic studies have suggested that higher intake of added sugar is associated with cardiovascular disease (CVD) risk factors."[16] Few prospective studies have examined the association of added sugar intake with CVD mortality, according to Quanhe Yang, a senior scientist in the CDC's division for heart disease and stroke prevention.

Unfortunately, regulation of sugar in the United States is not in the immediate future. Ben Tinker, CNN medical news senior producer, writes in his blog, "Despite our changing scientific understanding and a growing body of evidence on sugar overconsumption as an independent risk factor in chronic disease, sugar regulation remains an uphill battle in the United States. This is contrasted by the increased frequency of regulation abroad, where 15 countries now have taxes on sugar-sweetened beverages."[17, 18]

In that same blog, Tinker quotes Laura Schmidt, a professor of health policy in the School of Medicine at the University of California at San Francisco: "Sin taxes, whether on tobacco, alcohol, or sugar-laden products, are popular because they are easy to enforce and generate revenue, with a well-documented evidence base supporting their effectiveness for lowering consumption."[19]

One final thought comes from Kristin Kirkpatrick, MS, RD, LD, director of Wellness Nutrition Services at the Cleveland Clinic Wellness Institute: "Sugar is the true silent killer. Move over salt and hypertension, you've got competition. Sugar, as it turns out, is just as much of a silent killer."[20]

Appendix

Help with Your Food Safety Questions and Complaints

These government and nonprofit food safety agencies and organizations have answers to most of your questions about food safety issues.

Center for Food Safety (CFS)

www.centerforfoodsafety.org Tel: 202.547.9359. CFS is on top of many food safety issues, but its main work is helping protect human health and the environment by curbing the use of harmful food production technologies and by promoting organic and other forms of sustainable agriculture. CFS also educates consumers concerning the definition of organic food and products.

Center for Media and Democracy

http://www.prwatch.org/cmd Tel: 608.260.9713. This is one of my favorite sites, and its initials are familiar to me. CMD is a boutique investigative research and reporting group with a demonstrated capacity to break major news stories and highlight the work of advocates. They would love to hear from you, especially if you have a hot tip about a food safety issue.

Center for Science in the Public Interest (CSPI)

www.cspinet.org 202.332.9110. CSPI has been around for about 40 years and has long been a key player in educating the public about health and food issues as well as maintaining a strong counter to the food industry's powerful influence on public opinion and public policies. Founder Michael Jacobson, PhD, has been a familiar face in Washington helping to pass laws benefiting the consumer. He is the former commissioner of the U.S. FDA and publishes the award-winning *Nutrition Action Healthletter* for some 900,000 subscribers in the United States and Canada.

Centers for Disease Control and Prevention (CDC)

www.cdc.gov Tel: 404.639.3311. This may be the starting point for your questions. Here you'll find an abundance of information covering almost every disease about which you may have questions, and not just about foodborne illnesses. The search engine within the CDC website takes you to every corner of this important U.S. government agency.

Consumer Federation of America (CFA)

www.consumerfed.org Tel: 202.387.6121. Established in 1968, this nonprofit consumer organization is a research, education, and service organization producing investigative reports and analysis on a variety of subjects before federal and state regulatory agencies and state legislatures. "Not-Ready-To-Eat: How the Meat and Poultry Industry Weakened Efforts to Reduce Listeria Food Poisoning," is a terrific CFA report, which I have mentioned in this book.

Cruise Ship Inspections

http://wwwn.cdc.gov/InspectionQueryTool/InspectionSearch.aspx. Planning a cruise? The U.S. Centers for Disease Control and Prevention provides a quick way to read the latest inspection report regarding the ship on which you are booked. The CDC conducts the inspections under its Vessel Sanitation Program. You can use the site's "Advanced Search" option to reveal the ship's history of violations.

Foodborne Outbreak Online Database (Food)

http://wwwn.cdc.gov/foodborneoutbreaks/. The Centers for Disease Control and Prevention allows you to search its database for information on foodborne outbreaks reported to the CDC. You can search by year, location of the outbreak, and by the etiology (genus only).

Food and Drug Administration (FDA)

http://www.fda.gov Tel: 1.888.463.6332. The FDA is responsible for the safety of our food through regulations, inspections, and enforcements. All foods except meat and poultry fall under the giant umbrella of the FDA (issues concerning eggs are shared with the USDA). The FDA also has regulatory and enforcement authority for drugs, medical devices, radiation-emitting products, vaccines, blood and biologics, cosmetics, tobacco products, and certain aspects of animal and veterinary issues. (Unless it has changed, when you open the FDA's website, the first item you see is a large search bar. That's the best way to get around.)

Food Safety News (FSN)

http://www.foodsafetynews.com Tel: 206.407.2201. Food safety attorney Bill Marler assembled a team of experienced journalists who stay on top of breaking news concerning recalls, outbreaks, and closures 24/7. Updates of current news are posted on the website throughout the day. FSN usually comes up with the latest food safety news before any other site.

Institute of Food Technologists (IFT)

http://www.ift.org Tel: 800.438.3663. This is the largest food science organization in the world, encompassing almost 18,000 members worldwide as of 2012. IFT is an international, nonprofit organization dedicated to the advancement of food science and technology.

Journal of the American Medical Association (JAMA)

https://jama.jamanetwork.com/journal.aspx Tel: 1.800.262.2350. This is probably the most prestigious and widely circulated journal about all phases of medicine and related issues including food safety. Published continuously since 1883, some of the most critically acclaimed articles about food safety have appeared first in *JAMA*.

Local and State Health Departments

Your local government provides health inspection services at restaurants, hotels, hospitals, schools, nursing homes, street vendors, shopping center kiosks, fairs, festivals, and other food service facilities not covered by the FDA or the USDA. Inspection reports are public record and can be viewed and copies purchased under your state Open Records Law or the federal Freedom of Information Act. Report any possible violation of food safety laws to your local health department.

Mercy for Animals

https://www.mercyforanimals.org Tel: 866.632.6446. The Mercy for Animals website clearly states its mission: "We serve as a voice for animals through proactive consumer education initiatives, cruelty investigations, corporate outreach, and legal advocacy. Over 95% of the cruelty to animals in the United States occurs at the hands of the meat, dairy and egg industries which confine, mutilate, and slaughter over nine billion land animals each year." The website provides information about investigations, upcoming events, and how you can become active in the organization.

National Academy of Sciences (NAS)

http://www.nasonline.org Tel: 202.334.2000. Established in 1863, the National Academy of Sciences is a private, nonprofit society of distinguished scholars charged with providing independent, objective advice to the nation on matters related to science and technology. More than 500 members of NAS have won Nobel Prizes. The academy has published numerous reports and recommendations on food safety issues.

National Institutes of Health (NIH)

http://www.nih.gov Tel: 301.496.4000. As part of the U.S. Department of Health and Human Services, the NIH is the nation's medical research agency—making important discoveries that improve health and save lives. A search of the NIH database will produce numerous reports on a variety of food safety issues.

National Toxicology Program (NTP)

http://ntp.niehs.nih.gov Tel: 919.541.3419. Here is where you can learn about the 80,000 chemicals registered for use in the United States. Many of the chemicals are found in our food and elsewhere in our daily lives. The mission of NTP is to evaluate agents of public health concerns by developing tools of modern toxicology and molecular biology.

Pew Health Group

http://www.pewtrusts.org/default.aspx Tel: 215.575.9050. This independent nonprofit organization focuses on global research and public policy. The group operates as a nonpartisan, nongovernmental organization dedicated to serving the public. Pew addresses a variety of issues, from threats to the nation's food supply to the healthfulness of food served to schoolchildren. Numerous reports on food safety, food additives, and Pew's campaign to preserve the effectiveness of antibiotics by phasing out the overuse and misuse of the drugs in food animal production are available. A weekly newsletter is offered at no cost.

The USDA Meat and Poultry Complaint Hotline

Tel: 1.888.674.6854. This hotline is staffed by food safety experts Monday through Friday from 10:00 a.m. to 4:00 p.m. Eastern time. Issues concerning eggs are handled by both the USDA and the FDA. For all other complaints or problems with food, you can contact the FDA in your state. A list of the phone numbers for Consumer Complaint Coordinators is posted at the FDA website.

Local and State Health Departments

Your local government provides health inspection services at restaurants, hotels, hospitals, schools, nursing homes, street vendors, shopping center kiosks, fairs, festivals, and other food service facilities not covered by the FDA or the USDA. Inspection reports are public record and can be viewed and copies purchased under your state Open Records Law or the federal Freedom of Information Act. Report any possible violation of food safety laws to your local health department.

Notes

INTRODUCTION

1. "Nearly Three-Quarters of Americans Looking to Government for More Food Safety Oversight," Harris Interactive: Harris Polls, New York, February 5, 2014.

1. BIOTERRORISM, CYBER ATTACKS

1. David Heymann, "Terrorist Threats to Food—Guidance for Establishing and Strengthening Prevention and Response Systems," *Food Safety Issues*, World Health Organization, May 2008.

2. Barton Gellman, "Al Qaeda near biological, chemical arms production," *Washington Post*, March 23, 2003.

3. Katherine McIntire Peters, "Growing Threat," *Government Executive*, June 1, 2003.

4. James Risen with Don Van Natta Jr., "Threats and responses: Terror network; plot to poison food of British troops is suspected," *New York Times*, January 24, 2003.

5. Anthony Kimery, "The Threat of Bioterrorism and the Ability to Detect It," *Homeland Security Today*, US, December 29, 2010.

6. Caroline Smith DeWaal, "Rising Imports, Bioterrorism, and the Food Supply," *Food and Drug Law Journal*, vol. 59, no. 3, 2004.

7. Ibid., 3.

8. Peter Chalk, "Agroterrorism—What Is the Threat and What Can Be Done About It?" RAND Corporation, May 2, 2004.

9. Ibid., 9.

10. Robert Mueller, "Protecting Food from Terrorists," Speech at the International Conference on Agroterrorism in Kansas City, Missouri, May 2005; *Christian Science Monitor*, August 17, 2005.

11. "Risk Assessment for Food Terrorism and Other Food Safety Concerns," CFSAN/Office of Regulations and Policy. II. Risk Assessment, A. Hazard Identification. http://seafood.oregonstate.edu/.pdf%20Links/
Rish%20Assessment%20for%20Food%20Terrorism%20and%20Other%20Food%20Safety%20Concerns.pdf, October 7, 2003.

12. Ali S. Khan, Alexandra M. Levitt, and Michael J. Sage, "Biological and Chemical Terrorism: Strategie Plan for Preparedness and Response," *Morbidity and Mortality Weekly Report*, April 21, 2000/49$$04, 1–14.

13. Ibid., 13.

14. "Terrorist Threats to Food," *Food Safety Issues*, World Health Organization, May 2008.

15. Robert Turesky, "The Chemcial Terrorism of Food," Wadsworth Center of the New York State Department of Health, 2005.

16. President Obama Address to the United Nations General Assembly, September 21, 2011.

17. Khan et al., "Biological and Chemical Terrorism."

18. "Ready or Not—Chemical Terrorism Project," Association of Public Health Laboratories (APHL), "Catching Up with Bioterrorism Readiness," p. 10. http://www.aphl.org/AboutAPHL/publications/Documents/PHPR_2003July_Ready-or-Not-Findings-and-Recommendations-of-the-APHL-Chemical-Terrorism-Project.pdf.

2. FOOD IMPORTS

1. Andrew Bridges, "Imported food rarely inspected," *USA Today*, April 16, 2007.

2. Y. Buisson, J. L. Marie, and B. Davoust, "These Infectious Diseases Imported with Food," Science.gov, November 12, 2013.

3. Gabrielle Cosel, "Focus On: Food Import Safety—Food Safety Modernization Act," PEW Health Group, Center for Science in the Public Interest, 2011.

4. "Multistate Outbreak of Human Salmonella montevideo Infections (Final Update)," U.S. Centers for Disease Control and Prevention, May 4, 2010.

5. "Focus On: Food Import Safety, Food Modernization Act," PEW Health Group. March 2008.

6. Stephanie Kwisnek, "FDA Warns of Salmonella Risk with Cantaloupes from Agropecuaria Montelibano," United States Food and Drug Administration News Release, March 22, 2008.

7. "Melamine Pet Food Recall," U.S. Food and Drug Administration, October 7, 2009.

8. "T.M. Kovacevich International, Inc. Recalls Cantaloupe Because of Possible Health Risk," FDA website, March 25, 2008.

9. "Focus On: Food Import Safety—Food Safety Modernization Act. Recommendations for Improving Import Safety," PEW Health Group, 2010.

10. "A Decade of Dangerous Food Imports from China," *Food & Water Watch*, June 8, 2011.

11. Meagan Cline, "Tainted and Fake Honey from China," EthicalFoods.com, October 2013.

12. "Sweet deal? Maybe not. beware of honey sold in stores. It may not be honey," *Monroe News*, November 27, 2011.

13. "Harsh Sentences Handed Down for Chinese Food Safety Violations," *Food Production Daily*, February 10, 2012.

14. Grace Ng, "China Food Safety: From Bad Eggs to Foul Fowl," *Asia News Network,* January 1, 2013.

15. Cao Yin and Luo Wangshu, "Rotting meat used to make illegal oil," *China Daily News*, April 4, 2012.

16. Wang Hongyi, "Food safety tops public's concerns," *China Daily*, August 21, 2008.

17. Ibid.

18. Ibid., 5.

19. Wang Hongyi, "KFC supplier used excessive additives in chicken feed," *China Daily*, December 21, 2012.

20. Ibid., 5.

21. Fred Gale and Jean C. Buzby, "Imports from China and Food Safety Issues," *ERS Report Summary*, July 2009, USDA.

22. *Interpol Operation Opson* (Interpol.int, December 6, 2011).

23. Ibid., 7.

24. Hannah Gould, "CDC Research Shows Outbreaks Linked to Imported Foods Increasing—Fish and Spices the Most Common," Press Release, U.S. Centers for Disease Control and Prevention, March 14, 2012.

25. Helena Bottemiller, "Investigation: USDA Quietly Eliminated 60 Percent of Foreign Meat Inspections—Agency Also Lacks Foreign Audit Transparency," *Food Safety News*, www.foodsafetynews.com, November 1, 2012.

26. Ibid., 6.

27. Ibid., 7.

28. Ibid.

29. Steven Reinberg, "Better Safeguards Needed for Imported Food, Drugs: Report," *Health Day*, April 4, 2012.

30. Jim Avila, Kevin Dolak, and Carrie Gann, "Is Your Orange Juice Safe? FDA Says Carbendazim Causes No Safety Concern," ABC's Good Morning America, February 3, 2012.

31. Matt Paish, "Exclusive: World Food Safety Expert on Challenges in Delivery Food Safety in a Global Food Chain," *Australian Food News*, May 14, 2012.

32. Colin Thurston, "Is Europe Outpacing the U.S. in Traceability?" *Food Quality & Safety,* August/September 2013.

33. Jeff Gerth and Tim Weiner, "Tainted imports—Special report: Imports swamp U.S. food-safety efforts," *New York Times*, Archives section, September 29, 1997.

3. PRODUCE

1. "MDP—Program Overview," Science and Laboratories section of the Agricultural Marketing Service of USDA, last updated June 19, 2013.

2. Ibid., 1.

3. Garance Burke, "Obama Budget Cuts Bacteria Testing for Produce," *Huffington Post,* May 23, 2014.

4. Ibid., 2.

5. Ibid.

6. Michele Simon, "A Budget Cut Only the Produce Industry Could Love," EatDrinkPolitics.com, February 28, 2012.

7. Hank Campbell, "Federal Microbiological Data Program for Food Testing Shut Down," *Science 2.0*, January 11, 2013.

8. Ibid., 3.

9. "Salmonella Infection," Mayo Clinic, April 5, 2014.

10. "Salmonellosis," National Center for Emerging and Zoonotic Infectious Diseases, U.S. Centers for Disease Control and Prevention, November 16, 2009.

11. Ibid., 4.

12. "Multistate Outbreak of Listeriosis Linked to Whole Cantaloupes from Jensen Farms, Colorado," U.S. Centers for Disease Control and Prevention, August 27, 2012.

13. Ibid., 5.

14. "FDA Announces Recall of Cantaloupe by Chamberlain Farms of Owensville Indiana; Farm's Cantaloupe May Be One Source of Contamination in Multi-State Outbreak of Salmonellosis," FDA News Release, August 22, 2012.

15. "Delmonte packaged cantaloupes recalled due to possible Salmonella contamination," *Examiner*, April 2, 2011.

16. "Multistate Outbreak of Salmonella litchfield Infections Linked to Cantaloupe (Final Update)," U.S. Centers for Disease Control and Prevention, April 2, 2008.

17. Ibid., 5.

18. "Investigation Announcement: Multistate Outbreak of E. coli O157:H7 Infections Linked to Romaine Lettuce," U.S. Centers for Disease Control and Prevention, December 7, 2011.

19. Ibid., 5.

20. "Optimizing Produce Food Safety Is 'Simply Good Business'—PricewaterhouseCooper," *Bites*, Kansas State University, April 20, 2012.

21. "Multistate Outbreak of Salmonella Typhimurium Infections Linked to Peanut Butter, 2008–2009 (Final Update)," U.S. Centers for Disease Control and Prevention, May 11, 2010.

22. Ibid., 6.

23. "Letter to Sunland Inc. Concerning Suspension of Food Facility Registration; Notice of Opportunity for Hearing," U.S. Food and Drug Administration, November 26, 2012.

24. Jonel Aleccia, "FDA Names Taylor Farms as Source in Parasite Outbreak," NBC News, August 2, 2013.

25. Ibid., 7.

26. "Investigation of an Outbreak of Salmonella Saintpaul Infections Linked to Raw Alfalfa Sprouts," U.S. Centers for Disease Control and Prevention, May 8, 2009.

27. Ibid.

28. "Salmonella Newport Outbreak Linked to Alfalfa Sprouts," PritzkerLaw, May 28, 2010. http://foodpoisoning.pritzkerlaw.com/archives/cat-sprouts-salmonella-outbreak.html.

29. "Why Raw Sprouts May Be the Riskiest Food in Your Grocery Store," HuffPost-Food, *Huffington Post*, June 11, 2011.

30. "Papaya Food Poisoning: CDC Update on Salmonella Agona Outbreak," CDC report, "Food Poisoning Law Blog," July 27, 2011.

31. Ibid., 8.

32. "Multistate Outbreak of Salmonella Braenderup Infections Associated with Mangoes (Final Update)," U.S. Centers for Disease Control and Prevention, October 11, 2012.

33. Ibid.

34. Ibid., 8.

35. Ibid., 9.

36. Theresa Eisenman, "FDA Proposes 'Action Level' for Arsenic in Apple Juice, "FDA News Release, U.S. Food and Drug Administration, July 12, 2013.

37. Langan Denhard and Brandel France de Bravo, "Arsenic and Lead in Our Juice (and You Thought Poisoned Apples Were Only in Fairy Tales!)," National Center for Health Research, 2012.

38. "FDA Data Show Arsenic in Rice, Juice, and Beer," *Consumer Reports*, February 6, 2014.

39. John A. Painter et al., "Attribution of Foodborne Illnesses, Hospitalizations, and Deaths to Food Commodities by Using Outbreak Data, United States, 1998–2008," U.S. Centers for Disease Control and Prevention, March 2013.

40. Ibid., 10.

41. Drew Goodman, *Cultivating a Movement: Organic & Sustainable Farming* (University of California-Santa Cruz Digital Collections, Earthbound Farm, 2014).

42. Chip Carter, "Retailers Choosing Costs and Profits Over Safety, Major Industry Executive Says," *Food Policy & Safety*, April 7, 2014.

43. Ibid., 11.

44. Ibid.

45. Ibid.

46. Chip Carter, "Industry Executive Says Retailers Shortchange Safety, Put Profits First," About.com. Food Policy & Safety, May 31, 2013.

4. POULTRY

1. Tony Corbo, "USDA's Failure to Stop Contaminated Chicken Goes Far Beyond the Government Shutdown," Common Dreams, October 10, 2013.

2. Ibid., 1.

3. "Food Safety Update at Foster Farms' Livingston Plant," Press Room, Foster Farms, January 8, 2014. http://fosterfarms.com/about/press/press_release.asp?press_release_id=165.

4. Fred Pritzker, "Foster Farms Plant Closed by USDA: Cockroaches Found, Says Salmonella Lawyer," Food Poisoning Law Blog, January 9, 2014.

5. "What Is Salmonellosis?" Centers for Food Safety and Prevention, last updated April 5, 2012.

6. Ibid., 2.

7. "The High Cost of Cheap Chicken," *Consumer Reports*, February 2014.

8. David Pierson, "Costco unsure how cooked chicken was tainted in Salmonella outbreak," *Los Angeles Times,* October 14, 2013.

9. Ibid., 2.

10. Dr. Tom Frieden, "Antibiotic Resistance Threats in the United States, 2013," U.S. Centers for Disease Control and Prevention, April 23, 2013.

11. Ibid., 2.

12. Alon Galor, "City council supports antibiotic restriction," *The Brown Daily Herald*, February 25, 2014.

13. Stephanie Strom, "F.D.A. bans three arsenic drugs used in poultry and pig feeds," *New York Times*, October 1, 2013.

14. Ibid., 4.

15. James Greiff, "What Was Arsenic Doing in Our Chicken, Anyway?" *Bloomberg View,* October 10, 2013.

16. Ibid., 4.

17. Steve Holt, "Finally: American Chickens Will No Longer Be Fed Arsenic," *Take Part*, October 2, 2013.

18. Keeve E. Nachman et al., "Roxarsone, Inorganic Arsenic, and Other Arsenic Species in Chicken: A U.S.-Based Market Basket Sample," *Environmental Health Perspectives*, National Institutes of Health, 2013.

19. Keeve E. Nachman et al., "Poultry Drug Increases Levels of Toxic Arsenic in Chicken Meat," Johns Hopkins Center for a Livable Future, May 11, 2013.

20. Chris Hunt, "The Arsenic in Your Chicken," *Huff Post Green*, May 13, 2013.

21. David Wallinga, "Playing Chicken—Avoiding Arsenic in Your Meat," Institute for Agriculture and Trade Policy, Food and Health Program, April 2006.

22. Ibid.

23. Ibid., 6.

24. "Russia, U.S. to hold poultry talks in Moscow," *Ria Novosti*, January 19, 2010.

25. Anna Ghosh, "Food & Water Watch Exposes USDA Inspection Staffing Shortages," *Food & Water Watch*, February 10, 2014.

26. Ibid., 7.

27. Amanda Palleschi, "Government Executive: USDA 'Playing Chicken with Food Safety,' Protesters Charge," *Food Whistleblower*, http://www.foodwhistleblower.org, April 2, 2012.

28. Walker Foley, "Doo Doo Chicken: The New Pink Slime," *Food & Water Watch*, April 2, 2012.

29. Jim Avila, "USDA to Let Industry Self-Inspect Chicken," ABC News, April 18, 2012.

30. Al Almanza, "USDA to Let Industry Self-Inspect Chicken," interviewed on ABC News and published in the *Huffington Post*, April 18, 2012.

31. Martha Neil, "'Pink Slime' Beef Producers Sue ABC, Diane Sawyer, USDA Microbiologist and Others, Seek $1.2B," *ABA Journal,* September 13, 2012.

32. Marion Nestle, "Toxic Chicken Is the New Pink Slime," *Food Politics*, www.foodpolitics.com, April 9, 2012.

33. Dana Milbank, "Budget cuts as back-door deregulation," *Washington Post*, April 2, 2012.

34. Ron Nixon, "Plan to let poultry plants inspect birds is criticized," *New York Times*, April 4, 2012.

35. Ibid., 9.

36. Caroline Smith DeWaal, "Playing Chicken: The Human Cost of Inadequate Regulation of the Poultry Industry," *Food Safety News*, March 1996.

37. "Indian Ban on Imports of U.S. Poultry Sparks WTO Dispute," International Centre for Trade and Sustainable Development, *Bridges* vol. 16, no. 9, March 7, 2012.

38. "Fecal Contamination in Retail Chicken Products," Report from the Physicians Committee for Responsible Medicine, April 2012.

39. Susan Levin, "Physicians Committee for Responsible Medicine Survey," PCRM 2012 Study of Poultry, 2012.

40. Shua J. Chai et al., "Salmonella Enterica Serotype Enteritidis: Increasing Incidence of Domestically Acquired Infections," *Oxford Journals, Clinical Infectious Diseases*, vol. 54, issue suppl. 5, S488-497, 2012.

41. Rod Dreher, "Chicken Melamine," *The American Conservative*, September 9, 2013.

42. Peter Collignon et al., "Human Deaths and Third-Generation Cephalosporin use in Poultry, Europe," U.S. Centers for Disease Control and Prevention, August 2013.

43. "Public Health Dispatch: Outbreak of Listeriosis—Northeastern United States," Public Health Dispatch, *Morbidity and Mortality Weekly Report*, U.S. Centers for Disease Control and Prevention, October 25, 2002.

44. Tom Johnston, "China Puts Clamps on Jennie-O Plant," *Meatingplace*, August 12, 2013.

45. Valentina Pop, "EU 'Will Not Compromise' on Food Safety in US Trade Pact," *EUObserver*, February 12, 2014.

46. "EU 'Will Not Compromise' on Food Safety in US Trade Pact," *Europa NU,* February 20, 2014.

5. EGGS

1. Elizabeth Dahl and Caroline Smith DeWaal, "Scrambled Eggs—How a broken food safety system let contaminated eggs become a national food poisoning epidemic," Center for Science in the Public Interest, May 1997.

2. Gary Farber, "Which Came First: The Regulation or the Egg?" *Obsidian Wings*, September 22, 2010.

3. Ibid., 2.

4. Nancy H. Bean et al., "Surveillance for Foodborne-Disease Outbreaks—United States, 1988–1992," *Morbidity and Mortality Weekly Report*, Centers for Food Safety and Prevention, October 25, 1996.

5. Henry J. Holcomb, "They Run But They Can't Hide Florio, Fork in Hand, Takes on Egg Police," *The Inquirer*, Trenton Bureau, January 18, 1992.

6. Caroline Smith DeWaal, "Scrambled Eggs: How a Broken Food Safety System Let Contaminated Eggs Become a National Food Poisoning Epidemic," Center for Science in the Public Interest, May 1997.

7. Ibid., 2.

8. Ibid., 3.

9. Cynthia Galli, Angela Hill, and Rym Momtaz, "McDonald's Target Dump Egg Supplier After Investigation," ABC 20/20, November 18, 2011.

10. Ibid.

11. Elizabeth A. Waltrip, "Inspections, Compliance, Enforcement, and Criminal Investigations," FDA letter, re: Sparboe Farms/Prairie Complex, November 16, 2011.

12. Nathan Runkle, "Where Does Your Egg McMuffin Come From?" ABC News Investigation, November 18, 2011.

13. Paul Walsh, "Federal agents swarm Sparboe Farms," *Minneapolis Star Tribune*, January 8, 2013.

14. "Egg Titan and Son Charged in 2010 Salmonella Outbreak," NBC News, May 21, 2014.

15. Smith DeWaal, "Scrambled Eggs."

16. "Country report on the Swedish experience relating to the control of Salmonella," Food and Agriculture Organization of the United Nations, Agenda item 4.2a, January 28–30, 2002.

17. Lyndsey Layton, "Unsafe eggs linked to U.S. failure to act," *Washington Post*, December 11, 2010.

18. Ibid., 6.

19. Nadia Arumugam, "Why American Eggs Would Be Illegal in a British Supermarket, and Vice Versa, *Forbes*, October 25, 2012.

20. Ibid., 6.

21. Ibid., 7.

22. "Djehuty Ma'at-Ra, "Asinity of Egg Consumption," Dhealth Store, August 15, 2012. https://www.dhealthstore.com/index.php/articles/health-wellbeing/asininity-of-consumption.html Dherbs.com.

23. "Research finds egg yolks almost as bad as smoking," *Western News*, Western University, Canada, August 13, 2012.

24. Janice Stanger, "The Perfect Formula Diet: How to Lose Weight and Get Healthy Now With Six Kinds of Whole Foods," Blog of Janice Stanger, PhD, February 3, 2013.

25. "Bad Eggs Show Need for Better Food Safety Enforcement," *Star-Ledger* (New Jersey), August 29, 2010.

6. BEEF AND PORK

1. Charles E. Hanrahan, "The European Union's Ban on Hormone-Treated Meat," Congressional Research Service Reports, RS20142, updated December 19, 2000.

2. "What's in that pork? We found antibiotic-resistant bacteria and traces of a veterinary drug," ConsumerReports.org, January 2013.

3. Ibid.

4. Major Vic Harris et al., "Crisis communication strategies, analysis, case study: Jack in the box E. coli crisis," U.S. Department of Defense, no date provided, http://www.ou.edu/deptcomm/dodjcc/groups/02C2/team%20members.htm.

5. "Multi-State Salmonella Outbreak Linked to Taco Bell," MarlerClark, Attorney at Law, http://www.marlerclark.com/salmonella-taco-bell-texas-oklahoma/ (no date listed in the article).

6. Michael Moss, "The Burger That Shattered Her Life," *New York Times*, October 3, 2009.

7. Bob Edlin, "US data show high percentages of supermarket meat contains antibiotic-resistant bacteria," *AgScience,* The Nziahs Blog, April 18, 2013.

8. Christine Grillo, "The Science Is Clear: Antibiotic Resistance and Food Animal Production," Center for a Livable Future, 2014.

9. Shelly Burgess, "FDA takes steps to protect public health," U.S. Food and Drug Administration, News Release, April 11, 2012, last updated, May 13, 2013.

10. Barbara Kessler, "Public Health Advocates Criticize FDA for not Stopping Meat Industry's Rampant Antibiotic Use," PA Home Page, http://www.pahomepage.com/story/public-health-advocates-criticize-fda-for-not-stop/d/story/vt4ydCdG_UmJXuTaG5CCww, February 17, 2014.

11. Ibid.

12. Ibid.

13. Andrew Gunther, "Would you like extra Ractopamine with your pork, sir?" *Huffington Post*, Huff Post Food, December 5, 2012.

14. Helena Bottemiller, "Dispute over drug in feed limiting U.S. meat exports," Food & Environment Reporting Network, January 25, 2012.

15. Gunther, "Would You Like Extra Ractopamine With Your Pork, Sir?"

16. Anastasia Garina, "Russia throws poisonous meat back to US," Pravada.ru, English version, November 12, 2012.

17. Ibid.

18. Kathy Lally and Will Englund, "Russia fumes as U.S. Senate passes Magnitsky law aimed at human rights," *Washington Post*, Europe section, December 6, 2012.

19. Codexalimentarius, International Food Standards World Health Organization (WHO). http://www.codexalimentarius.org.

20. Tommy Dean, "Why 160 countries say 'no' to US meat," *Veg News*, March 14, 2013.

21. Ibid., 2.

22. "Codex Alimentarius: Statement by the EU on Ractopamine," Europa—Health and Consumers, http://ec.europa.eu/food/fs/ifsi/eupositions/cac/cac_index_en.html, July 2012.

23. Ibid., 6.

24. "Rampant mislabeling of beef in Korea," *Food Navigator-Asia*, October 14, 2013.

25. "When science becomes business when business runs governments," *America's Food Industry*, November 1, 2013.

26. "Rampant mislabeling of beef in Korea."

27. Dean, "Why 160 countries say 'No.'"

28. "Bovine growth hormone," *Food &Water Watch,* http://www.foodandwaterwatch.org/food/foodsafety/dairy/.

29. "Recombinant bovine growth hormone (rBGH)," American Cancer Society, February 18, 2011.

30. Ibid.

31. "Examples of Audit and Investigative Work for Goal," Office of Inspector General, Semiannual Report to Congress, U.S. Department of Agriculture, p.1, December 2013.

32. Andrew MacLeod, "Gov't moving to keep farm disease outbreaks secret," *The Tyee,* Vancouver, British Columbia, May 15, 2012.

33. "Rampant animal cruelty at California slaughter plant," Humane Society of the United States, January 30, 2008.

34. Ted Genoways, "Gagged by big ag: Horrific abuse. Rampant contamination. And the crime is . . . exposing it?" *Mother Jones*, July/August 2013.

35. "Undercover investigation documents pig abuse at Tyson supplier," Humane Society of the United States, May 8, 2012.

36. James Barragan, "Meatpacking firms reach settlement on animal cruelty charges," *Los Angeles Times*, November 27, 2013.

37. Monica Eng, "Humane Society files complaint against Smithfield Foods for animal welfare claims," *Chicago Tribune*, November 2, 2011.

38. Anna West, "HSUS exposes inhumane treatment of pigs at Smithfield," Humane Society of the United States, December 15, 2010.

39. Wayne Pacelle, "HSUS exposes inhumane treatment of pigs at Smithfield," Humane Society of the United States, December 15, 2010.

40. Bill Haslam, "Tenn. Governor Haslam vetoes anti-whistleblower bill," Humane Society of the United States, May 13, 2013.

41. Ibid.

42. "Anti-whistleblower bills hide factory-farming abuses from the public," Humane Society of the United States, January 7, 2014.

43. "Eating with our eyes closed," *New York Times*, Opinion Pages, April 9, 2013.

44. "Animal cruelty: Attacking the messenger," *Boston Globe*, Editorials, April 15, 2013.

45. Bruce Campion-Smith, "Ottawa to allow slaughterhouses to process already dead animals," TheStar.com, Canada, May 14, 2012.

46. "Azodicarbonamide: Another reason to avoid most bread," Examiner.com, June 4, 2009.

47. Meredith Melnick, "Why lovin' the McRib isn't heart smart," *Time*, Nutrition Section, October 27, 2011.

48. Ibid.

49. Whet Moser, "The invention of the McRib and why it disappears from McDonald's," *Chicago Magazine*, October 25, 2011.

50. *Vessel Sanitation Program's Operations Manual* (Atlanta, GA: Centers for Disease Control and Prevention, 2005), p. 17.

51. Mike McGraw, "Beef's raw edges, building bigger cattle: An industry overdose," *Kansas City Star*, December 2012.

52. Ibid.

53. Ibid.

54. "Outbreaks linked to tenderized/marinated steaks originating in the United States," compilation of FSIS generated data. p. 34592 (Federal Register Vol. 78 No. 111/Monday, June 10, 2013/Proposed Rules, Table 2— June 10, 2013).

55. Pia A. Ang, "Philippines' food and agricultural import regulations and standards—Narrative gain report," U.S. Department of Agricultural Services, December 31, 2012.

56. Demetrios Marantis, "Sanitary and Phytosanitary Measures," SPS Report from the United States Trade Representative, March 2013.

57. Mark Post, *Taste Test: Lab-Grown Hamburger Short on Flavor*, Maastricht University, The Netherlands August 5, 2013.

7. MILK

1. Interview with Julie Riggs for "Real Stories of the Dangers of Raw Milk," U.S. Centers for Disease Control and Prevention, January 24, 2011.

2. Ibid.

3. Ibid.

4. Interview with Kalee Prue for "Real Stories of the Dangers of Raw Milk," U.S. Centers for Disease Control and Prevention, January 24, 2011.

5. Interview with Mary McGonigle-Martin for "Real Stories of the Dangers of Raw Milk," U.S. Centers for Disease Control and Prevention, January 24, 2011.

6. Ibid.

7. "Raw (Unpasteurized) Milk: Trying to Decide about Raw Milk?" U.S. Centers for Disease Control and Prevention, February 25, 2013.

8. Health Advisory, "Raw Milk and Raw Dairy Products—Risk and Recommendations," California Department of Public Health Advisory, February 18, 2014.

9. "Majority of Dairy-Related Disease Outbreaks Linked to Raw Milk," U.S. Centers for Disease Control and Prevention February 21, 2012.

10. "Raw Milk Always a Risk: Study of 2012 Family Cow Food Poisoning," *Campylobacter Outbreak Bulletin*, May 4, 2013.

11. "Notes from the field: Recurrent outbreak of Campylobacter, JeJuni infections associates with a raw milk dairy—Pennsylvania," August 30, 2013, 62(34): 702–702; *Morbidity and Mortality Weekly Report*. April–May 2013.

12. Karen Rowan, "Raw Milk Sickened Scores Despite Inspections," *Live Science*, May 1, 2013.

13. Carla Gillespie, "Organic Pastures Outbreak Is Fifth Raw Milk Outbreak This Year," *Food Poisoning Bulletin*, May 13, 2012.

14. Rowan, "Raw Milk Sickened Scores."

15. Ibid.

16. "Questions and Answers—Raw Milk," U.S. Food and Drug Administration, March 1, 2007, last update November 1, 2011.

17. Gillespie, "Organic Pastures Outbreak."

18. "Summary of the Foundation Farm raw milk-associates E. coli O157:H7 outbreak," Oregon Health Authority, Public Health Division, Office of Disease Prevention & Epidemiology, Acute and Communicable Disease Prevention, 2012.

19. Ibid., 5.

20. Linda Larsen, "Raw milk E. coli outbreak sickens 12 in Missouri," *Food Poisoning Bulletin*, April 13, 2012.

21. "Milk Safety," Missouri Department of Health and Senior Services, http://health.mo.gov/safety/foodsafety/pdf/safemilk.pdf.

22. "Summary of the Foundation Farm raw milk-associated E. coli O157."

23. Jon Van, "'85 Salmonella outbreak largest ever, study says," *Chicago Tribune*, December 11, 1987.

24. "Salmonella outbreak is traced," *New York Times,* April 17, 1985.

25. Blythe Bernhard, "E. coli outbreak in Missouri doesn't dissuade raw milk fans," *St. Louis Post-Dispatch*, April 13, 2012.

26. Ibid., 6.

27. "Questions and Answers—Raw Milk."

28. "The Dangers of Raw Milk: Unpasteurized Milk Can Pose a Serious Health Risk," U.S. Food and Drug Administration, June 17, 2013.

29. Kim Palmer, "Raw milk sickens more than widely reported, study says," *USA Today*, December 11, 2013.

8. SEAFOOD

1. Jordan Bailey, "The FDA Only Inspects 1–2% of Imported Seafood from China," Economy in Crisis—America's Economic Report Daily, March 19, 2014.

2. "Import Guidance," Seafish.org, August, 2010.

3. "Justification of Estimates for Appropriations Committees," U.S. Food and Drug Administration, 2013.

4. "Outside the U.S.," Fishwatch—U.S. Seafood Facts, September 6, 2013.

5. Ibid., 2.

6. "Marine Toxins," U.S. Centers for Disease Control and Prevention, October 12, 2005.

7. Vernon E. Ansdell, "Food Poisoning from Marine Toxins," U.S. Centers for Disease Control and Prevention, August 1, 2013.

8. Ibid., 3.

9. Ibid.

10. Vernon E. Ansdell, "Food Poisoning from Marine Toxins," The United States Centers for Disease Control and Prevention, August 1, 2013.

11. Ibid.

12. Martha Iwamoto et al., "Epidemiology of Seafood-Associated Infections in the United States," Introduction, *Clinical Microbiology Reviews*, American Society for Microbiology, April 2010.

13. Ibid., 4.

14. Ibid.

15. "Foodborne Illness Surveillance, Response, and Data Systems," U.S. Centers for Disease Control and Prevention, January 14, 2014.

16. *Vibrio* Illness (Vibriosis): Vibrio parahaemolyticus," U.S. Centers for Disease Control and Prevention, October 21, 2013.

17. "Study: Oceana Study Reveals Seafood Fraud Nationwide," Oceana.org. February 21, 2013.

18. Sen. John McCain, "The Fishy Deal on Catfish," Politico.com, June 7, 2013.

19. "Eartheasy," Sustainable Seafood, http://eartheasy.com/eat_sustainable_seafoods.htm.

20. Mindy Pennybacker and P. W. McRandle, "Guide to Which Fish Are Safe to Eat," Organic Consumers Association, February 24, 2004.

21. Leslie Beck, "The safest fish to eat? Follow this rule, new study suggests," *The Globe and Mail,* Toronto, August 10, 2012.

22. "Fish Consumption Advisories," U.S. Environmental Protection Agency, www.water.epa.gov/scitech/swguidance/fishshellfish/fishadvisories/index.cfm.

9. DELI DANGERS

1. "FSIS Comparative Risk Assessment for Listeria monocytogenes in Ready-to-eat Meat and Poultry Deli Meats Report," U.S. Department of Agriculture, Food Safety and Inspection Service, May 2010.

2. Benjamin J. Silk et al., "Vital Signs: Listeria Illnesses, Deaths, and Outbreaks—United States, 2009–2011," *Morbidity and Mortality* Weekly Report, U.S. Centers for Disease Control and Prevention, June 7, 2013.

3. Michael B. Batz, Sandra Hoffmann, and J. Glenn Morris Jr., "Ranking the Risks—The 10 Pathogen-Food Combinations with the Greatest Burden on Public Health," Emerging Pathogens Institute, University of Florida, 2011.

4. "Interagency Retail Listeria Monocytogenes Risk Assessment," Public Meeting, U.S. Department of Health and Human Service's Food and Drug Administration/Center for Food Safety and Applied Nutrition, U.S. Department of Agriculture's Food Safety and Inspection Service, June 23, 2009.

5. Martin Wiedman, "Using Risk Assessment to Design Effective Intervention—Case Study: Listeria and Deli Meat," Cornell University College of Agriculture and Life Sciences, Department of Food Science, September 2013.

6. "Interagency Risk Assessment: Listeria monocytogenes in Retail Delicatessens, The Interagency Retail Listeria monocytogenes Risk Assessment Workgroup," U.S. Department of Agriculture, September 2013.

7. Ibid., 2.

8. Jennifer C. McEntire, "Microwaving Deli Meat: The Only Real Food-Safe Option?" The Acheson Group, May 30, 2013.

9. Ibid.

10. Laura Landro, "Informed Patient: Danger in the Deli? Listeria Risks Go Beyond Cantaloupe," *Wall Street Journal* Health Blog, October 3, 2011.

11. Adelina Espat, "Deli Meat and Bacon: Charisse's Challenge," University of Texas MD Anderson Center, July 2013.

12. "Processed Meats Too Dangerous for Human Consumption," Institute for Natural Healing, World Cancer Research Fund, updated May 22, 2013.

13. Mary Ellen Herndon, "Deli Meat and Bacon: Charisse's Challenge," University of Texas MD Anderson Cancer Center, MD Anderson website, July 2013.

14. Sami L. Gottlieb et al., "Multistate Outbreak of Listeriosis Linked to Turkey Deli Meat and Subsequent Changes in US Regulatory Policy," *Clinical Infectious Diseases,* Vol. 42, Issue 1, August 7, 2005.

15. "Colorectal Cancer, Facts & Figures, 2011–2013," American Cancer Society, 2011.

16. Brittany Risher, "Decoding the Deli Counter," *Women's Health*, January 30, 2014.

17. "Pregnant or Older? Be Safe with Ready-to-Eat Meats," U.S. Centers for Disease Control and Prevention, May 2011, http://www.cdc.gov/media/matte/2011/05_listeriapregnant.pdf.

18. "Red and Processed Meats and Cancer Prevention," World Cancer Research Fund, 2004.

19. Sabine Rohrmann et al., "Meat Consumption and Mortality—Results from the European Prospective Investigation into Cancer and Nutrition 2013," BMC Medicine 2013.

20. Lilia McFarland, "Louisiana Firm Recalls Cooked Meat, Poultry, and Deli Products Due to Possible Listeria Monocytogenes Contamination," Press Release, U.S. Food and Drug Administration, April 12, 2013.

21. Letter from Chris Waldrop, Director, Food Policy Institute of the Consumer Federation of America, to the U.S. Food and Drug Administration, re: Docket No. FDA-2008-D-0058 April 14, 2008.

22. Carol Tucker Foreman and Christopher Waldrop, "Not Ready-to-Eat: How the Meat and Poultry Industry Weakened Efforts to Reduce Listeria Food Poisoning," Consumer Federation of America, December 2000, 33, 34.

23. Ibid.

24. Ibid., 8.

25. Ibid.

10. OUTBREAKS, ILLNESSES, AND DEATHS

1. Paul S. Mead et al., "Food-Related Illness and Death in the United States," *Emerging Infectious Diseases*, vol. 5, no. 5, September–October 1999.

2. Jim Gorman, "The 10 dirtiest foods you're eating," *Men's Health*, 2012.

3. Ibid.

4. Joe Whitworth, "Top 6 deadliest foodborne pathogens - Salmonella ranks as the pathogen most linked to deaths after a decade-long Centers for Disease and Control and Prevention (CDC) surveillance report," Food Quality News, September 23, 2013.

5. Chrissy Christoferson testimony, U.S. Food and Drug Administration hearing, Washington, DC, July 25, 2013.

6. Ibid.

7. "KFC told to pay $8.3 million to Australian girl poisoned by Twister wrap," NBC News, April 27, 2012.

8. Hon. Stephen Rothman, New South Wales Supreme Court Justice, New South Wales Supreme Court, 2005.

9. Robert V. Tauxe, "Emerging Foodborne Diseases: An Evolving Public Health Challenge," *Emerging Infectious Diseases*, vol. 3, no. 4, October–December 1997, 429.

10. Madeline Drexler, "Animal Farms," PBS Frontline.

11. Clifford Mintz, "The Top 10 Foodborne Illness Outbreaks in the US," ehealthforum.com, July 11, 2011.

12. "Epidemiologic Notes and Reports Update: Milk-borne Salmonellosis—Illinois," *Morbidity and Mortality Weekly Report*, U.S. Centers for Disease Control and Prevention. April 1985.

13. "Salmonella outbreak is traced," *New York Times*, April 17, 1985.

14. Swati Agiwal and Hamid Mohtadi, "Risk Mitigating Strategies in the Food Supply Chain," University of Minnesota, Department of Applied Economics, Selected Paper prepared for presentation at the American Agricultural Economics Association Annual Meeting, Orlando, Florida, July 27–29, 2008.

15. "Investigation Announcement: Multistate Outbreak of Salmonella Enteritidis Infections Linked to Restaurant Chain A," U.S. Centers for Disease Control and Prevention, January 19, 2012.

16. Chris Morran, "Taco Bell Named in Salmonella Enteritis Outbreak," *Consumerist*, February 2, 2012.

17. Ryan Jaslow, "Taco Bell tied to 2011 Salmonella outbreak that sickened 68," CBS News, February 2, 2012.

18. "Taco Bell lettuce suspected in E.coli outbreak," CNN Money, December 13, 2006.

19. Phyllis Entis, "Taco Bell Named in Multi-State Salmonella Outbreak," efoodalert.wordpress.com, February 1, 2012.

20. Benjamin J. Silk et al., "Vital Signs: Listeria Illnesses, Deaths, and Outbreaks—United States, 2009–2011," *Morbidity and Mortality Weekly Report,* U.S. Centers for Disease Control and Prevention, June 4, 2013.

21. Ibid., 6.

22. Mintz, "Top 10 Foodborne Illness Outbreaks."

23. Dennis D'Amico, "Incidence, Ecology, and Fate of Target Foodborne Pathogens in the Cheesemaking Continuum," Dissertation, Dennis D'Amico, University of Vermont, October 2008.

24. Ryan J. Foley, "U.S. charges egg company, 2 execs in 2010 outbreak," ABC News, May 21, 2014.

25. Peter Perl, "Poisoned package," *Washington Post*, January 16, 2000.

26. Peter Perl, "Listeria fear forces recall of hot dogs," *Washington Post*, March 26, 2000.

27. "Listeria outbreak rattles USDA," Iowa Public Television, October 18, 2002.

28. Douglas Karas, "FDA Confirms Listeria monocytogenes on Jensen Farms' Rock Ford-brand Cantaloupes," U.S. Food and Drug Administration, September 19, 2011.

29. Scott Bronstein and Dew Griffin, "Third-deadliest U.S. food outbreak was preventable, experts say," CNN Health, May 3, 2012.

30. David Gombas, "Guidance on Environmental Monitoring and Control of Listeria for the Fresh Produce Industry," United Fresh Food Safety & Technology Council, American Mushroom Institute, 2013.

31. "Diseases and Conditions—E. Coli," Mayo Clinic, July 28, 2011.

32. "E. coli (Escherichia coli)—General Information," Centers for Disease Control and Prevention, November 10, 2011, Updated August 3, 2012.

33. Anthony E. Fiore, "Hepatitis A Transmitted by Food, "Division of Viral Hematitis, Centers for Disease Control and Prevention, February 11, 2004.

34. "Veggies and Fruit are the Top Food Poisoning Culprits," Food Poison Journal, January 31, 2006.

35. Barbara K. Hecht, and Frederick Hecht, "Hepatitis A Was in Green Onions," Medicine-Net.com (no date provided)

36. "Fatal Foodborne Clostridium Perfringens at a State Psychiatric Hospital—Louisiana, 2010," Morbidity and Mortality Weekly Report, Centers for Disease Control and Prevention, August 17, 2012.

37. Sophie Borland and Emine Sinmaz, "'They sent her home and she lay in my arms dying': Husband's anger at hospital and pub after his wife dies from suspected Christmas Day food poisoning," Mail Online, London Daily Mail, January 3, 2013.

38. "Clostridium Perfringens," January 29, 2014.

39. "Rotavirus," Centers for Disease Control and Prevention," May 12, 2014.

40. Ibid.

41. Ibid.

42. Ibid.

43. Ibid.

44. "Norovirus is so common the Health District doesn't bother keeping stats on it," *Las Vegas, CityLife*, January 9, 2013.

45. "Norovirus," Centers for Disease Control and Prevention, October 30, 2013. http://www.cdc.gov/norovirus/.

46. Alexandra Sifferlin, "The 13 Worst Norovirus Outbreaks on Cruise Ships," *Time*, January 27, 2014.

47. Samantha Henry, Associated Press, "Cruise ship passengers recall days of misery," *USA Today*, January 29, 2014.

48. Brenda Goodman, "Norovirus Outbreak Traced to Reusable Grocery Bag—Study Underscores How Easily Norovirus Can Spread," WebMD Health News, May 9, 2012. http://archive.today/NFvPK.

49. "Parasites—Toxoplasmosis (Toxoplasma infection)," U.S. Centers for Disease Control and Prevention, January 10, 2013.

50. "What are the risks of toxoplasmosis during pregnancy?" National Health Service, (NHS) UK, March 5, 2014.

51. Betty Bowles, Nelda Coleman, and Lauren Jansen, "Toxoplasmosis," p. 7, Midwestern State University. http://faculty.mwsu.edu/nursing/lauren.jansen/toxoplasmosis.pdf.

52. "Cyclosporiasis Outbreak Investigations—United States, 2013 (Final Update)," U.S. Centers for Disease Control and Prevention," December 2013.

53. Ibid., 11.

54. Sydney Lupkin, "Cyclospora victim: 'I found myself in tears a lot of the time'," Good Morning America, ABC-TV News, August 2, 2013.

55. Ibid.

56. "FDA Investigates Multistate Outbreak of Cyclosporiasis," U.S. Food and Drug Administration, November 21, 2013.

57. W.O.K. Grabow, "Enteric Hepatitis Viruses—Hepatitis A Virus," World Health Organization, 1983.

58. Jorgen Schlundt, "Deliberate Contamination of Food: Recent Concern, Old Problem," Food Safety Threats—International Coordination, Addressing Foodborne Threats to Health: Policies, Practices, and Global Coordination: Workshop Summary, NCBI, National Institutes of Health, 2006.

59. Benedetto Terracini, ed., *Toxic Oil Syndrome, Ten Years of Progress,* World Health Organization—Europe, 2004.

60. Ashton Acton, ed., *Alkali Metals—Advances in Research and Application,* Ch.1, p. 98, ScholarlyEditions, Atlanta, GA, 2013.

61. Susan Klasing, "Evaluation of Potential Health Effects of Eating Fish from Selected Water Bodies in the Northern Sierra Nevada Foothills," *Nevada, Placer, and Yuba Counties Guidelines for Sport Fish Consumption*, p. 18, December 2003.

11. FOOD TAMPERING AND FOOD FRAUD

1. Iva Cheung, "10 Notorious Cases of Product Tampering," Listverse.com, December 27, 2010, http://listverse.com/2010/12/27/10-notorious-cases-of-product-tampering/.

2. Marc L. Ostfield, "Food Defense: The Vital Role of International Collaboration," Remarks by Marc L. Ostfield, Senior Advisor for Bioterrorism, Biodefense, and Health Security, U.S. Department of State at the Biennial Meeting of the National Center for Food Protection and Defense (NCFPD) at Chaska, Minnesota, June 28, 2007.

3. "Risk Assessment for Food Terrorism and Other Food Safety Concerns," CFSAN/Office of Regulations and Policy, October 7, 2003, http://seafood.oregonstate.edu/.pdf%20Links/Risk%20Assessment%20for%20Food%20Terrorism%20and%20Other%20Food%20Safety%20Concerns.pdf.

4. LeeAnne Jackson, "Overview of FDA's Food Defense Activities," Center for Food Safety and Applied Nutrition, U.S. Food and Drug Administration, January 26, 2012.

5. Ostfield, "Food Defense."

6. Michael Arndt, "Girl Scouts putting bad year behind," *Chicago Tribune*, February 3, 1985.

7. Alan Hoeting, "History of the U.S. Food and Drug Administration," Transcript of a taped oral history, U.S. Food and Drug Administration, pp. 28–31, April 21, 1999.

8. Steve Lohr, "Baby-food makers confront British contamination scare," *New York Times*, May 2, 1989.

9. Ibid.

10. Ibid., 3.

11. Clyde Haberman, "The great candy caper leaves all Japan atwitter," *New York Times*, World section, July 2, 1984.

12. Cheung, "10 Notorious Cases."

13. "Risk Assessment for Food Terrorism."

14. Ostfield, "Food Defense."

15. "Terrorism: Chemical Terrorism," Canadian Security Intelligence Service, Jewish Virtual Library, 1994.

16. "Annual Report FY 2000," U.S. Department of the Interior, U.S. Fish and Wildlife Service, Division of Law, 2000.

17. Monika Maria Lucia Freitas Dos Santos, "Defeating the Dragon: Heroin Dependence Recovery," Thesis, University of South Africa, Department of Psychology, June 2006.

18. Cheung, "10 Notorious Cases."

19. Ibid., 4.

20. Maria Glod, "Boy charged with food tampering," *Washington Post*, Virginia edition, May 10, 2007.

21. Kevin Martin, "Sentence handed Calgary food saboteur justified, appeal court rules," *Calgary Sun*, November 26, 2013.

22. Keith Nunes, "Nestle CEO calls horse meat scandal 'unforgivable'," *Food Business News*, February 26, 2013.

23. Alex Wang, "Food safety in China, or is that rat meat in my lamb?" *Legal Planet*, BerkeleyLaw UCLA Law, May 23, 2013.

24. Stephen Castle and Doreen Carvajal, "Counterfeit food more widespread than suspected," *New York Times*, June 26, 2013.

25. J. C. Moore, J. Spink, and M. Lipp, "Development and application of a database of food ingredient fraud and economically motivated adulteration from 1980 to 2010," *Journal of Food Science,* April 2012.

26. Hal Weitzman, "Four accused in US over tainted cheese," *Financial Times,* April 20, 2012.   http://www.ft.com/cms/s/0/e2fcb6dc-8a4c-11e1-93c9-00144feab49a.html#axzz33QEVc2IN.

27. Fauna, "Discarded Food Waste Slop Recycled into Cheap Cooking Oil," ChinaSmack, October 16, 2009.

28. Moore et al., "Development and application of a database."

29. "Crackdown on Fraudulent Food Labels Urged—CSPI Exposes Some of the Most Misleading Ingredient Claims," Center for Science in the Public Interest, October 27, 2005.

30. Ibid., 9.

31. Ibid., 11.

12. FOODS WE EAT, OTHERS WON'T

1. Charles W. Schmidt, "Organic Chicken Has Much Less Arsenic," *Environmental Health Perspectives,* 2012.

2. Paige Tomaselli, "FDA Admits Chicken Meat Contains Arsenic," Center for Food Safety, EcoWatch/News Investigation, May 8, 2013.

3. David Wallinga, "FDA Ignores Toxic Arsenic in Animal Feed," Agriculture and Trade Policy (IATP) Center for Food Safety website, May 1, 2013.

4. "Maryland Children's Environmental Health Progress Report," Maryland Environmental Health Network, January 17, 2013.

5. Kate Schneider, "The ancient lost city of Shi Cheng lies deep underwater," news.com.au, February 20, 2014.

6. "Singapore," One World Nations online, 2014, http://www.nationsonline.org/oneworld/singapore.htm.

7. Scott William, "Wake Up America and Read the Label Next Time," Scribd.com, 2013, http://www.scribd.com/doc/207122033/Wake-Up-America-and-read-the-label-next-time-you-buy-something.

8. Sen. Charles E. Schumer, "Schumer Reveals: Toxic, cancer-causing chemical that Subway sandwich chain voluntarily removed from their bread this week can still be found in scores of other fast food products; calls on FDA to ban chemical in foods nationwide," website of Sen. Charles E. Schumer, U.S. senator for New York, February 10, 2014.

9. Ibid., 3.

10. Charles E. Schumer, News Release, February 10, 2014.

11. Ibid., 3.

12. Ibid.

13. "Where does the FDA stand on the use of Azodicarbonamide?" Examiner.com, February 26, 2014.

14. "Everything Added to Food in the United States (EAFUS)," U.S. Food and Drug Administration, April 23, 2013.

15. Susan Donaldson James, "Kraft Agrees to Take Yellow Dye Out of Mac and Cheese," ABC News Good Morning America, October 31, 2013.

16. Ibid., 4.

17. Ibid.

18. Bernard Weiss, "Synthetic Food Colors and Neurobehavioral Hazards: The View from Environmental Health Research," *Environmental Health Perspectives,* National Institutes of Health, U.S. Department of Health and Human Services, September 16, 2011.

19. Sarah Kobylewski and Michael F. Jacobson, "CSPI Says Food Dyes Pose Rainbow of Risks—Cancer, Hyperactivity, Allergic Reactions," Center for Science in the Public Interest, June 29, 2010.

20. Ibid.

21. Heather Brodie Perry, "Petition to FDA from Heather Brodie Perry," Petition to Dr. Bernard A. Schwetz, DVM, PhD, Acting Principal Deputy Commissioner, Dockets Manage-

ment Branch, Food and Drug Administration, from Heather Brodie Perry, East Bridgewater, MA 02333, August 3, 2001.

22. J. H. Weisburger, "The 37-year history of the Delaney Clause," PubMed.gov, U.S. Library of Medicine, National Institutes of Health, February 1996.

23. Maciej Fita, "Some of Our Food Is Banned in Europe but for Sale in the U.S?" *Igozen*, August 22, 2013, http://www.igozen.com/did-you-know-some-of-our-food-is-banned-in-europe-but-for-sale-in-the-u-s/.

24. Susanna Kim, "11 Food Ingredients Banned Outside the U.S. That We Eat," ABC News report, June 26, 2013.

25. "10 American Foods that Are Banned Elsewhere," North Texas Wellness Center, November 21, 2013.

26. Ibid., 7.

27. Ibid.

28. Ibid.

29. "Eat This, Not That," *Men's Health*, 2013.

30. "Butylated Hydroxyanisole," *Report on Carcinogens*, 12th edition (2011), National Toxicology Program, Department of Health and Human Services.

31. "Natural Astaxanthin—The Distinct Differences between Natural and Synthetic Astaxanthin," Well Wise, August 2000.

32. Amy Cadora, "Ten U.S. Foods that are Banned in Other Countries," The Norwex Purpose in Action, September 16, 2013.

33. Ibid.

34. Hope Warshaw et al., "Fat Replacers: Their Use in Foods and Role in Diabetes Medical Nutrition Therapy," *DiabetesCare*, July 31, 1996.

35. Kim, "11 Food Ingredients Banned."

36. Melissa Dittman, "Protecting Children from Advertising," American Psychological Association, *Monitor on Psychology,* vol. 35, no. 6, Print version p. 58, June 2004.

13. UNWELCOME CRITTERS IN OUR FOODS

1. Eric Berger, "Top 10 grossest food defects the FDA deems safe for humans," *Houston Chronicle*, May 18, 2011.

2. Ibid., 1.

3. David L. Lewis et al., "Interactions of Pathogens and Irritant Chemicals in Land-Applied Sewage Sludges (Biosolids)," BMC Public Health, BioMedCentral, June 28, 2002.

4. Dave L. Lewis, et al., "Interactions of pathogens and irritant chemicals in land-applied sewage sludges (biosolids). United States National Library of Medicine, National Institutes of Health, 2002; 12(4):409–23.

5. "Laws and Regulations," U.S. Environmental Protection Agency, 2014, http://www2.epa.gov/laws-regulations.

6. Rebekah Wilce, "Under Pressure, Whole Foods Agrees to Stop Selling Produce Grown in Sewage Sludge," PR Watch, January 16, 2014.

7. Sarah Klein, "Gross Ingredients In Processed Foods," *Huffington Post*, May 14, 2012.

8. "Defect Levels Handbook—The Food Defect Action Levels," United States Food and Drug Administration, February 2005.

14. GMOS—GENETICALLY MODIFIED ORGANISMS

1. Andrew Kimbrell, "'Agent Orange' corn: Biotech only winner in chemical arms race as herbicide resistant crops fail," *Huffington Post*, February 22, 2012.

2. Ibid., 1.

3. "Time Is Running Out to Keep Hundreds of Millions of Pounds of Toxic Herbicide Off American Fields and Out of Our Environment," Center for Food Safety, 2014.

4. "EPA Set to Approve Increased Use of Toxic 2,4-D on Dow's 'Agent Orange' Crops," Center for Food Safety, May 1, 2014.

5. Ibid., 1.

6. "'Frankenfood' Fear: The GMO Debate," NewsChannel 5, WTVF-TV, November 22, 2013.

7. Joe Pizzomo Jr., "Genetically Modified Foods: Just Say No!" WebMD, Integrative Medicine and Wellness, November 20, 2007.

8. "Labeling Around the World," Just Label It, 2014, http://justlabelit.org/right-to-know/labeling-around-the-world/.

9. Kate Snipes and Carol Kamau, "Kenya Bans Genetically Modified Food Imports," Foreign Agricultural Service, U.S. Department of Agriculture, November 27, 2012.

10. "Biotechnology Project," Center for Science in the Public Interest, April 2012.

11. Ibid., 3.

12. Ibid.

13. Ibid., 4.

14. Ibid.

15. "Benefits of GM Food," University of California-Santa Cruz, 2014, http://classes.soe.ucsc.edu/cmpe080e/Spring05/projects/gmo/benefits.htm.

16. "Are Biotech Foods Safe to Eat?" WebMD, 2014.

17. Edison de Mello, "What's the big deal about genetically-modified organisms?" *HuffPost Healthy Living*, September 12, 2013.

18. Ibid., 7.

19. Ibid., 6.

20. Amy Dean, and Jennifer Armstrong, "Genetically Modified Foods," American Academy of Environmental Medicine, May 8, 2009.

21. "CDC Study of Unexplained Dermopathy," U.S. Centers for Disease Control and Prevention.

22. Elaine Watson, "Judge: 'There is a gaping hole in the current regulatory landscape for "natural" claims and GMOs,'" Food Navigator—USA.com, June 18, 2013.

23. Arjun Walla, "Scientists Discover Bt Toxins Found in Monsanto Crops Damage Red Blood Cells," Collective-evolution.com, May 11, 2013.

24. Ibid., 6.

25. Arjun Walla, "Scientists Discover Bt Toxins Found in Monsanto Crops Damage Red Blood Cells," Collective-Evolution, May 11, 2013.

26. Ibid., 7.

27. Ibid.

28. Ibid., 8.

29. Hank Schultz, "Advocate: People get ready, there's a non GMO train a comin'," Food Navigator-USA.com, August 8, 2013.

30. "Biotechnology Project," Center for Science in the Public Interest, April 2012.

31. Ibid., 9.

32. Ibid.

33. "Tomorrow Is Election Day ," EatDrinkVote.com, November 4, 2013.

34. Gary Langer, "Poll: Skepticism of Genetically Modified Foods," ABC News, June 19, 2013.

35. Jenny Hopkinson, "Lawmakers Ask Obama to Keep '07 GMO Labeling Promise," Politico Pro, TimiLi.com, January 16, 2014.

36. Andrew Kimbrell, "Citizen Petition Before the United States Food and Drug Administration," Center for Food Safety, 2011.

37. "Public Forces Food Industry to Sell Non-GMO Products, Ingredients," WordLoaf.com, 2014.

38. Richard Levick, "Are GMO-free Cheerios the first domino?" *Forbes*, January 9, 2014.

39. Jonathan Landsman, "The unpalatable truth: GMA wants GMOs kept secret," *Natural Health* 365, May 19, 2014.

40. Maggie Hannessy, "Food Industry Group Wants Permission to Label GMO Foods as 'Natural'," Food Navigator-USA.com, December 20, 2013.

41. Jon Entine, "GMO Science Denialists? ENSSER Challenges WHO, National Academy of Sciences on GM Safety," Genetic Literacy Project, May 27, 2014.

42. Amanda Cochron, "GMO Food Labeling: Inside the Controversy," CBS News, May 7, 2014.

43. Annie Gasparro and Leslie Josephs, "Whole Foods to Stop Selling Chobani Yogurt," *Wall Street Journal*, December 18, 2013.

44. Carey Gillam, "U.S. food companies find gong 'non-GMO' no easy feat," Reuters, February 18, 2014.

45. Ibid., 11.

15. GENERALLY RECOGNIZED AS SAFE

1. "How U.S. FDA's GRAS Notification Program Works," U.S. Food and Drug Administration, December 2005/January 2006.

2. Ibid.

3. Ashlee Kieler, "Potentially Harmful Chemicals Find Their Way Into Our Food Thanks to 56-Year-Old FDA Rule," *Consumerist*, April 7, 2014.

4. Tom Neltner and Maricel Maffini, "Generally Recognized as Secret: Chemicals Added to Food in the United States," Natural Resources Defense Council, April 2014.

5. Thomas G. Neltner et al., "Conflicts of Interest in Approvals of Additives to Food Determined to Be Generally Recognized as Safe Out of Balance," *Journal of the American Medical Association*, December 9, 2013.

6. Andrew M. Seaman, "Industry Influence Found in Food Additives," PEW Health Initiatives, August 7, 2013.

7. "Pew Initiative on Food and Biotechnology," The Pew Trusts, April 2004.

8. Ibid., 2.

9. Michael F. Jacobson, "Letter to the Food Standards Australia & New Zealand," Center for Science in the Public Interest, September 22, 2010.

10. http://www.mycoprotein.org

11. "FDA Should Strengthen Its Oversight of Food Ingredients Determined to Be Generally Recognized as Safe (GRAS)," U.S. Government Accountability Office, March 5, 2010.

12. Ibid.

13. Ibid.

14. Rita Jane Gabbett, "NRDC says GRAS list is a loophole for unsafe chemicals in food," *Meatingplace*, April 8, 2014.

15. "FDA Should Strengthen Its Oversight."

16. "Tentative Determination Regarding Partially Hydrogenated Oils; Request for Comments and for Scientific Data and Information," A Notice by the Food and Drug Administration on Federal Register, November 8, 2013.

17. Shelly Burgess, "FDA Takes Step to Further Reduce Trans Fats in Processed Foods," U.S. Food and Drug Administration, November 7, 2013.

18. Robert Chacanaca et al., Plaintiffs, v. The Quaker Oats Company, Defendant, No. C 10-0502 RS, United States District Court for the Northern District of California, San Jose Division, filed and decided October 14, 2010.

19. Gyorgy Scrinis, "The Trans-Fats Fiasco," *Huffington Post*, November 13, 2013.

20. Eric Decker, "The Impact and Consequences of Banning Trans Fatty Acids," Institute of Food Technologists, November 19, 2013.

21. Ibid., 7.

22. "FDA Proposes to Eliminate Artificial Trans Fat in Processed Foods," Institute of Food Technologists, *The Weekly*, November 13, 2013.

23. Rachael Rettner, "Will You Even Notice The Trans Fat Ban?" *HuffPost Healthy Living*, November 13, 2013.

16. BPA—BISPHENOL A

1. "Corporate Positions on BPA," Breast Cancer Fund, 2014.
2. Willi Eibner, "Greiner Packaging International 'BPA-free,'" News release, September 2013.
3. "BPA: What, When, Where, How, Why," Baum, Hedlund, Aristei, & Goldman, PC, consumer attorneys, 2014.
4. "Chemical Listed Effective April 11, 2013 as Known to the State of California to Cause Reproductive Toxicity: Bisphenol A (BPA)," Office of Environmental Health Hazard Assessment, State of California, April 2013.
5. "The Phenol & Acetone Sector Group," Petro Chemistry—Europe, http://www.petrochemistry.eu/about-petrochemistry/products.html?filter_id=17.
6. Leah Zerbe, "FDA: We won't ban BPA (for now)," *Rodale News*, March 30, 2012.
7. "Bisphenol A," Safer States, February 2013, http://www.saferstates.com/toxics_in_our_lives/chemicals_of_concern/BPA.html.
8. "Government Guidelines for the Safety & Dangers of Plastic Containers (Including Baby Bottles and Microwavable Bowls)," New Parents Network and U.S. Department of Health and Human Services, July 12, 2013.
9. "Bisphenol A (BPA)," National Institutes of Health, U.S. Department of Health and Human Services, May 22, 2014.
10. "Infant Feeding Module," Clinic Services Unit of the Texas Department of State Health Services, pp. 2–28. December 2012.
11. Gwynne Lyons, "The concerns about Bisphenol A (BPA) and recommendations for action. A CHEM Trust Position Paper, December 2010.
12. "Bisphenol A (BPA)."
13. "Bisphenol A (BPA)."
14. Sarah Yang, "BPA linked to thyroid hormone changes in pregnant women, newborns," Berkeley Research, University of California, October 4, 2012.
15. Ibid.,4.
16. Janet Gray, "State of the Evidence—The Connection between Breast Cancer and the Environment," Breast Cancer Fund, 2010.
17. Ibid.
18. Jim Avila, "BPA, Common Chemical, Affects Sex in Mice; Warning for Us?" Column by Lee Dye via World News, a television report on BPA, a chemical often used in plastics, altered the sexual patterns of California mice, say scientists, reported by Jim Avila, ABC News, February 15, 2013.
19. De-Kin Li et al., "Urine Bisphenol-A Level in Relation to Obesity and Overweight in School-Age Children," PloS One, U.S. National Library of Medicine, 2013.
20. "Bisphenol A," Diabetes and the Environment website, 2013, http://www.diabetesandenvironment.org/home/contam/bpa.
21. Jenni Spinner, "Doctors win $8m grant to look at BPA effects on babies," *Food Production Daily*, August 22, 2013.
22. Kara Kelber, "Consumers Union Applauds FDA Move to Ban BPA in Infant Formula Packaging," Consumers Union, July 11, 2013.
23. Ibid.

17. THE COTTAGE FOOD INDUSTRY AND YOUR KITCHEN

1. "Michigan Cottage Foods Information," Michigan Department of Agriculture and Rural Development, 2014.
2. Rachel Zemser, "No You Can't Sell Cottage Cheese Out of Your Cottage Food Operation," FoodProductDesign.com, April 30, 2013.

3. Rob Walsh, "Go Texan, Eat Local, Support Texas Cottage Food," *Texas Eats*, September 29, 2010.

4. Christopher Bedford, "Guest Editorial: Why We Need a Cottage Food Law," *Lansing Online News,* May 17, 2010.

5. Ibid., 2.

6. "Cottagefoods.org," Cottage Food laws, Florida, 2014.

7. Zemser, "No You Can't," 3.

8. Kirstin Kolpitcke, "Letter to Colorado Governor Brown, re: California Homemade Food Act, AB 1616," Legislative Representative, League of Cities August 31, 2012.

9. Ibid., 4.

10. "Check Your Steps," FoodSafety.gov. (no date provided)http://www.foodsafety.gov/keep/basics/

11. "Safe Cooking Temperatures," chart, Food and Drug Administration (no date provided) http://www.fda.gov/downloads/Food/FoodborneIllnessContaminants/UCM260394.pdf.

12. "Prize-Winning Poster," Health Education Council.

18. RESTAURANT FOOD

1. Ashlee Kieler, "Study Finds Produce, Restaurants Most Likely to Give Consumers Foodborne Illnesses," *Consumerist*, April 8, 2014.

2. William Lyon, "Managing German Cockroaches," Entomology Fact Sheet, NHE-3, Cooperative Extension Service, University of Illinois, April 1996.

3. "The German Roach," Interview with Donald Reierson at the University of California, Riverside, 1983.

4. Michael K. Rust statement to Charles M. Duncan, April 23, 2014.

5. Ed Bark, "Duncan does tasteful job with restaurant series," *Dallas Morning News*, February 7, 1983.

6. Interview with Dr. Ed Manning Washington, D.C., 1983.

7. Caroline Smith DeWaal and Elizabeth Dahl, "Dine at Your Own Risk—The Failure of Local Agencies to Adopt and Enforce National Food Safety Standards for Restaurants," Center for Science in the Public Interest, November 1996.

8. Ibid., 5.

9. Ibid.

10. Ibid., 6.

11. Ibid.

12. Ibid., 6.

13. "Preliminary Report: Foodborne Outbreak of Escherichia coli O157:H7 Infections from Hamburgers—Western United States, 1993," *Morbidity and Mortality Weekly Report*, U.S. Centers for Disease Control and Prevention, February 5, 1993.

14. "Hazard Analysis & Critical Control Points (HACCP)," U.S. Food and Drug Administration, July 5, 2013.

15. DeWaal and Dahl, "Dine at Your Own Risk," 7.

16. "Food Establishment Inspection Form," U.S. Food and Drug Administration, December 2003, http://www.foodprotect.org/media/guide/CFPFoodEstabInspFormCommFormApp-xA.pdf.

19. GOVERNMENT'S REPORT CARD

1. Leslie Pray and Ann Yaktine, *Managing Food Safety Practices from Farm to Table*, National Academies Press, 2009.

2. Rick Pendrous, "Closer scrutiny of US food imports promised," *Food Navigator-USA*, March 2, 2011.

3. "President's Food Safety Working Group," March 14, 2009, http://www.foodsafetyworkinggroup.gov/ContentLearn/HomeLearn.htm.

4. Ibid., 1.

5. Ibid.

6. Ibid.

7. Ibid.

8. "FDA to require imported food to be inspected at the source," Homeland Security newswire, September 4, 2013.

9. Anna Edney, "Food Risk Rises as Import Reliance Makes U.S. Safety Harder," Bloomberg.com, April 4, 2012.

10. "Policy Statement Database, Toward a Healthy, Sustainable Food System," American Public Health Association, November 6, 2007.

11. "Investigation Announcement: Multistate Outbreak of Salmonella Enteritidis Infections Linked to Restaurant Chain A," U.S. Centers for Disease Control and Prevention, January 19, 2012.

12. Steven Reinberg, "Better Safeguards Needed for Imported Food, Drugs: Report," Health Day, April 4, 2012.

13. Bill Marler, "Bill Marler Delivers Food Bank Safety Keynote," MarlerClark, Food Safety Attorneys at Law, June 1, 2012, www.marlerclark.com.

14. "2012 Annual Report: Opportunities to Reduce Duplication, Overlap and Fragmentation, Achieve Savings, and Enhance Revenue, GAO-12-342SP," U.S. Government Accountability Office, February 2012.

15. Ibid., 3.

16. Ibid., 4.

17. Sascha Haverfield, "Resources Must Keep Pace with FDA's Increasing Responsibilities to Patients and Consumers," Phrma.org, May 28, 2013.

18. Ibid., 4.

19. "FDA Budget Primer: Frequently Asked Questions," Alliance for a Stronger FDA, May 30, 2013.

20. *Center for Food Safety, et al., v. Margaret A. Hamburg, M.D.,* U.S. District Court, Northern District of California, No. C 12-4529 PJH, August 13, 2013.

21. Ibid., 5.

22. Gina Shaw, "Despite Delays in Implementation of FSMA, the Food Industry Moves Forward," *Food Quality & Safety*, December/January 2013.

23. "2011 Estimates of Foodborne Illness in the United States," U.S. Centers for Disease Control and Prevention, April 15, 2011.

24. Steve Benen, "House GOP targets food safety, WIC, nutrition aid," *Washington Monthly*, Political Animal blog, June 17, 2011.

EPILOGUE

1. Nancy Appleton, "141 Reasons Sugar Ruins Your Health (Just Kidding, It's 143)," http://www.nancyappleton.com.

2. Robert Lustig, "Sugar: The Bitter Truth," video lecture at the University of California San Francisco School of Medicine, May 26, 2009.

3. Ibid.

4. Art Carden, "Should We Regulate Sugar Like Alcohol or Tobacco?" *Forbes*, February 2, 2012.

5. William Coda Martin, "Refined Sugar—The Sweetest Poison of All," article posted in Global Healing Center, no date available, extracted from *Sugar Blues* by William Duffy (Padnor, PA: Chilton Book Company, 1975).

6. Ibid.

7. Jennifer Ashton, "Can Sugar Be Poisonous?" Jennifer Ashton's Twitter page, April 18, 2011, and CBS Early Show, April 18, 2011.

8. Dr. Mark Hyman, "Sweet poison: How sugar, not cocaine, is one of the most addictive and dangerous substances," *New York Daily News*, February 10, 2014.

9. Stephanie Johnson, "Houston, We Have a Problem: Sugar," Advocate Health Care, Health enews, September 30, 2013.

10. "A Little About Sugar," Healthy Lifestyle, Central Connecticut Senior Health Services website, November 1, 2013.

11. "Sugar: How Much Are You Eating?" Pure Performance Physical Training, July 4, 2013, http://www.pppt.com.au/category/news/.

12. Teya Skae, "The Harmful Effects of Sugar and Choosing Healthy Alternatives," Natural News, February 21, 2008.

13. Ibid.

14. "FDA Urged to Determine Safe Limits on High-Fructose Corn Syrup and Other Sugars in Soft Drinks," Center for Science in the Public Interest, February 13, 2013.

15. "Sugar Association Finds Opinion Piece Published in Nature Non-Scientific and Irresponsible," Sugar Association, February 2, 2012.

16. Quanhe Yang et al., "Added Sugar Intake and Cardiovascular Diseases Mortality among U.S. Adults," National Institutes of Health, PubMed.gov, U.S. National Library of Medicine, April 2014.

17. Ben Tinker, "Sugar Not Only Makes You Fat, It May Make You Sick," CNN Health, "The Chart" blog, February 3, 2014.

18. Ibid., 7.

19. Ibid.

20. Kristin Kirkpatrick, "10 Things You Don't Know About Sugar (And What You Don't Know Could Hurt You)," HuffPost Healthy Living, July 30, 2013.

Bibliography

"A Decade of Dangerous Food Imports from China." Food & Water Watch, June 8, 2011.

Acton, Ashton, ed. *Alkali Metals—Advances in Research and Application*, ScholarlyEditions, June 21, 2013 Ch. 1, p. 98, 2013.

Agiwal, Swati, and Hamid Mohtadi. "Risk Mitigating Strategies in the Food Supply Chain," University of Minnesota, Department of Applied Economics, Selected Paper prepared for presentation at the American Agricultural Economics Association Annual Meeting, Orlando, Florida, July 27–29, 2008.

Aleecia, Jonel. "FDA Names Taylor Farms as Source in Parasite Outbreak," NBC News, August 2, 2013.

Allen, Jonathan. "Bakers: Cottage Food Bill Unfair," Charleston, South Carolina, Patch, February 28, 2012.

Alliance for a Stronger FDA. "FDA Budget Primer: Frequently Asked Questions," May 30, 2013.

American Cancer Society. "Colorectal Cancer, Facts & Figures, 2011–2013."

———. "Recombinant Bovine Growth Hormone (rBGH)," February 18, 2011.

American Public Health Association. "Policy Statement Database, Toward a Healthy, Sustainable Food System," November 6, 2007.

Ang, Pia A. "Philippines' Food and Agricultural Import Regulations and Standards—Narrative Gain Report," U.S. Department of Agricultural Services, December 31, 2012.

Appleton, Nancy. "141 Reasons Sugar Ruins Your Health (Just Kidding, It's 143)," http://www.nancyappleton.com.

"Are Biotech Foods Safe to Eat?" WebMD, 201.

Arumugam, Nadia. "Why American Eggs Would Be Illegal in a British Supermarket, and Vice Versa," *Forbes,* October 25, 2012.

Avila, Jim, Kevin Dolak, and Carrie Gann. "Is Your Orange Juice Safe?: FDA Says Carbendazim Causes No Safety Concern," ABC's Good Morning America, February 3, 2012.

"Azodicarbonamide: Another Reason to Avoid Most Bread." Examiner.com, June 4, 2009.

Bailey, Jordan. "The FDA Only Inspects 1–2% of Imported Seafood from China," Economy in Crisis—America's Economic Report Daily, March 19, 2014.

Balter, S., H Hanson, L Kornstein, L Lee, V Reddy, S Sahl, F Stavinsky, New York City Department of Health and Mental Hygiene; M Fage, G Johnson, New York State Department of Health. J Bancroft, W Keene, Oregon Department of Human Services. J Koepsell, M Williams, Public Health Seattle and King County; K MacDonald, N Napolilli, J Hofmann, Washington State Department of Health. C Bopp, M Lynch, K Moore, J Painter, N Puhr, P Yu, Div of Foodborne, Bacterial, and Mycotic Diseases, National Center for Zoonotic, Vector-Borne, and Enteric Diseases (proposed), CDC. October 21, 2013.

Barragan, James. "Meatpacking firms reach settlement on animal cruelty charges," *Los Angeles Times*, November 27, 2013.

Bashsur, Ramona. "FDA and Regulation of GMOs," American Bar Association eSource, February 2013, vol. 9, no. 6.

Batz, Michael B., Sandra Hoffmann, and J. Glenn Morris Jr. "Ranking the Risks—The 10 Pathogen–Food Combinations with the Greatest Burden on Public Health," Emerging Pathogens Institute, University of Florida, 2011.

Baum, Hedlund, Aristei, and P.C. Goldman. "BPA: What, When, Where, How, Why," 2014.

Bean, Nancy H. "Surveillance for Foodborne-Disease Outbreaks—United States, 1988–1992," *Morbidity and Mortality Weekly Report*, Centers for Food Safety and Prevention, October 25, 1996.

Beck, Leslie. "The safest fish to eat? Follow this rule, new study suggests," *The Globe and Mail*, Toronto, August 10, 2012.

Bedford, Christopher. "Guest Editorial: Why We Need a Cottage Food Law," *Lansing Online News*, May 17, 2010.

"Benefits of GM Food." Genetically Modified Foods, article published online by the University of California-Santa Cruz, 2014, http://classes.soe.ucsc.edu/cmpe080e/Spring05/projects/gmo/benefits.htm.

Berger, Eric. "Top 10 grossest food defects the FDA deems safe for humans," *Houston Chronicle*, May 18, 2011.

"Bisphenol A." Safer States, February 2013. http://www.saferstates.com/toxics_in_our_lives/chemicals_of_concern/BPA.html.

Bottemiller, Helena. "Investigation: USDA Quietly Eliminated 60 Percent of Foreign Meat Inspections—Agency Also Lacks Foreign Audit Transparency," Food Safety News, http://www.foodsafetynews.com, November 1, 2012.

"Bovine Growth Hormone," Food and Water Watch, http://www.foodandwaterwatch.org/food/foodsafety/dairy/.

Breast Cancer Fund. "Corporate Positions on BPA," 2014.

Bridges, Andrew. "Imported food rarely inspected," *USA Today*, April 16, 2007.

Bronstein, Scott, and Drew Griffin. "Third-deadliest U.S. food outbreak was preventable, experts say," CNNHealth, May 3, 2012.

Burgess, Shelly. "FDA Takes Step to Further Reduce Trans Fats in Processed Foods," U.S. Food and Drug Administration, November 7, 2013.

Burke, Garance. "Obama Budget Cuts Bacteria Testing for Produce," *Huffington Post*, May 23, 2014.

Campbell, Hank. "Federal Microbiological Data Program for Food Testing Shut Down," Science 2.0, January 11, 2013.

Carden, Art. "Should We Regulate Sugar Like Alcohol or Tobacco?" *Forbes*, February 2, 2012.

Carter, Chip. "Industry Executive Says Retailers Shortchange Safety, Put Profits First," About.com Food Policy & Safety, May 31, 2013.

———. "Retailers Choosing Costs and Profits Over Safety, Major Industry Executive Says," Food Policy & Safety," April 7, 2014.

Center for Science in the Public Interest. "The 10 Riskiest Foods in America."

Center for Food Safety. "EPA Set to Approve Increased Use of Toxic 2,4-D on Dow's 'Agent Orange' Crops," 2014, http://www.centerforfoodsafety.org/issues/1044/rbgh/press-releases/3122/epa-set-to-approve-increased-use-of-toxic-24-d-on-dows-agent-orange-crops.

———. "Time is Running Out to Keep Hundreds of Millions of Pounds of Toxic Herbicide off American Fields and Out of Our Environment," 2014.

Center for Food Safety, et al., v. Margaret A. Hamburg, M.D., United States District Court, Northern District of California, No. C 12-4529 PJH, August 13, 2013.

Centers for Food Safety and Prevention. "What Is Salmonellosis?" last updated April 5, 2012.

Chacanaca, Robert v. The Quaker Oats Company, United States District Court for the Northern District of California, San Jose Division, No. C 10-0502 RS, filed and decided October 14, 2010.

Center for Science in the Public Interest. "Chemical Cuisine," 2014.

———. "CDC Report on Antibiotic Resistance Doesn't Deliver Action Steps to Address Food Safety, Says CSPI," September 16, 2013.

———. "Biotechnology Project." April 2012.

———. "Crackdown on Fraudulent Food Labels Urged—CSPI Exposes Some of the Most Misleading Ingredient Claims," October 27, 2005.

Cheung, Iva, "10 Notorious Cases of Product Tampering," ListVerse.com, http://listverse.com/2010/12/27/10-notorious-cases-of-product-tampering/, December 27, 2010.

Cline, Meagan. "Tainted and Fake Honey from China," Ethical Foods, October 2013.

Cochron, Amanda. "GMO Food Labeling: Inside the Controversy," CBS News, May 7, 2014.

"Codex Alimentarius: Statement by the EU on Ractopamine," Europa—Health and Consumers, http://ec.europa.eu/food/fs/ifsi/eupositions/cac/cac_index_en.html, July 2012.

Collignon, P., F., M. Aarestrup, R. Irwin, and S. McEwen. "Human deaths and third-generation cephalosporin use in poultry, Europe [letter]," *Emerg Infect Dis* [Internet]. 2013 Aug [date cited]. http://dx.doi.org/10.3201/eid1908.120681.

Cottagefoods.org. http://cottagefoods.org/food/granola/, July 21, 2013.

———. "Cottage Food Laws," Florida, 2014.

de Mello, Edison. "What's the Big Deal About Genetically-Modified Organisms?" *HuffPost Healthy Living*, September 12, 2013.

Dean, Amy, and Jennifer Armstrong. "Genetically Modified Foods," American Academy of Environmental Medicine, May 8, 2009.

Dean, Tommy. "Why 160 Countries Say 'No' to US Meat," *Veg News*, March 14, 2013.

"Delmonte packaged cantaloupes recalled due to possible Salmonella contamination," *Examiner*, April 2, 2011.

Denhard, Langan, and Brandel France de Bravo, "Arsenic and Lead in Our Juice (and You Thought Poisoned Apples Were Only in Fairy Tales!)" National Center for Health Research, 2012.

D'Amico, Dennis. "Incidence, Ecology, and Fate of Target Foodborne Pathogens in the Cheesemaking Continuum," Dissertation, Graduate College of the University of Vermont, October 2008.

DeWaal, Caroline Smith. "FDA Voluntary Guidance on Antibiotics Tragically Flawed," Center for Science in the Public Interest, April 11, 2012.

———. "Crisis and Consensus: Modernizing U.S. Food Safety Law," testimony before the House Appropriations Subcommittee on Agriculture, Rural Development, Food and Drug Administration, and Related Agencies, September 25, 2007.

———. "Scrambled Eggs: How a Broken Food Safety System Let Contaminated Eggs Become a National Food Poisoning Epidemic," Center for Science in the Public Interest, May 1997.

———. "Playing Chicken—The Human Cost of Inadequate Regulation of the Poultry Industry," Center for Science in the Public Interest, March 1996.

DeWaal, Caroline Smith, and Elizabeth Dahl. "Dine at Your Own Risk—The Failure of Local Agencies to Adopt and Enforce National Food Safety Standards for Restaurants," Center for Science in the Public Interest, November 1996.

Dos Santos, Monika Maria Lucia Freitas. "Defeating the Dragon: Heroin Dependence Recovery," University of South Africa, Department of Psychology, June 2006.

Dreher, Rod. "Chicken Melamine, *The American Conservative*, September 9, 2013.

Drexler, Madeline. "Animal Farms," PBS Frontline. An excerpt from *Secret Agents: The Menace of Emerging Infections* by Madeline Drexler, published by the Joseph Henry Press (2002).

———. "Secret Agent O157: The Evolution of a Killer," PBS Frontline, 2014.

"Eartheasy," Sustainable Seafood, http://eartheasy.com/eat_sustainable_seafoods.htm.

"Eat This, Not That," *Men's Health*, 2013.

"The U.S.D.A. Inspects Its Inspectors," *New York Times*, Opinion Pages, Editorial Board, June 17, 2013.

Edney, Anna. "Food Risk Rises as Import Reliance Makes U.S. Safety Harder," Bloomberg, April 4, 2012.

"Egg Titan and Son Charged in 2010 Salmonella Outbreak," NBC News, May 21, 2014.

Eisenman, Theresa. "FDA proposes 'action level' for arsenic in apple juice," *Chicago Tribune*, July 13, 2013.

Eng, Monica. "MDP—Program Overview," Agricultural Marketing Service of USDA, Science and Laboratoriessection, last updated June 19, 2013.

————. "Humane Society files complaint against Smithfield Foods for animal welfare claims," *Chicago Tribune*, November 2, 2011.

Entine, Jon. "GMO Science Denialists? ENSSER Challenges WHO, National Academy of Sciences on GM Safety," Genetic Literacy Project, May 27, 2014.

Entis, Phyllis. "Taco Bell Named in Multi-State Salmonella Outbreak," efoodalert.wordpress.com, February 1, 2012.

"Epidemiology of Infectious Diseases in Illinois." Department of Public Health, State of Illinois, 2003.

"Escherichia coli (E. coli) Infection." North Carolina Department of Health and Human Services, April 3, 2013.

Espat, Adelina. "Deli Meat and Bacon: Charisse's Challenge," University of Texas MD Anderson Center, July 2013.

"Facts and Ideas from Anywhere." PMC, National Institutes of Health, October 2013.

Farber, Gary. "EU 'Will Not Compromise' on Food Safety in US Trade Pact." Europa NU, February 20, 2014.

Fauna. "Discarded Food Waste Slop Recycled Into Cheap Cooking Oil," China Smack, October 16, 2009.

"FDA Data Show Arsenic in Rice, Juice, and Beer." *Consumer Reports*, February 6, 2014.

"FDA Proposes to Eliminate Artificial Trans Fat in Processed Foods." *The Weekly*, Institute of Food Technologists, November 13, 2013.

"FDA to require imported food to be inspected at the source." Homeland Security newswire, September 4, 2013.

Fita, Maciej. "Some of Our Food Is Banned in Europe but for Sale in the U.S?" *Igozen*, August 22, 2013.

"Fixing Food Safety: Protecting America's Food Supply from Farm-To-Fork; Focus On: Food Import Safety, Food Modernization Act," Pew Health Group. March 2008.

"Food Safety and Food Defense," BT Safety, 2014.

Foodsafeguru. "Update: 343,000+ pounds of Chilean Chicken with Dioxin Recalled," US Food Safety," August 15, 2013.

Foreman, Carol Tucker, and Christopher Waldrop. "Not Ready to Eat: How the Meat and Poultry Industry Weakened Efforts to Reduce Listeria Food-Poisoning," Consumer Federation of America, December 2004.

Frieden, Tom, MD, MPH. "Antibiotic Resistance Threats in the United States, 2013," U.S. Centers for Disease Control and Prevention, April 23, 2013.

Gale, Fred, and Jean C. Buzby. "Imports from China and Food Safety Issues," Economic Information Bulletin No. 52, U.S. Department of Agriculture, Economic Research Service, July 2009.

Galli, Cynthia, Angela Hill, and Rym Momtaz. "McDonald's, Target Dump Egg Supplier After Investigation," ABC News, November 18, 2011.

Galor, Alon. "City Council supports antibiotic restriction," *Brown Daily Herald*, February 25, 2014.

Gasparro, Annie, and Leslie Josephs. "Whole Foods to stop selling Chobani yogurt," *Wall Street Journal*, December 18, 2013.

Genoways, Ted. "Gagged by Big Ag—Horrific Abuse, Rampant Contamination," *Mother Jones*, July/August 2013 Issue.

Gerth, Jeff, and Tim Weiner. "Tainted imports, a special report: Imports swamp U.S. foodsafety efforts," *New York Times*, archives section, September 29, 1997.

Ghosh, Anna. "Food & Water Watch Exposes USDA Inspection Staffing Shortages," Food & Water Watch, February 10, 2014.

Gillam, Carey. "U.S. Food companies find going 'non-GMO' no easy feat," Reuters, February 18, 2014.

Gillespie, Carla. "Organic Pastures Outbreak is Fifth Raw Milk Outbreak This Year," *Food Poisoning Bulletin*, May 13, 2012.

Glod, Maria. "Boy charged with food tampering," *Washington Post*, Virginia edition, May 10, 2007.

Gombas, David. "Guidance on Environmental Monitoring and Control of Listeria for the Fresh Produce Industry," United Fresh Food Safety & Technology Council, American Mushroom Institute, 2013.

Goodman, Brenda. "Norovirus Outbreak Traced to Reusable Grocery Bag—Study Underscores How Easily Norovirus Can Spread," WebMD Health News, May 9, 2012.

Gorman, Jim. "The 10 Dirtiest Foods You're Eating," *Men's Health,* 2012.

Gottlieb, Sami L., et al. "Outbreak of Listeriosis Linked to Turkey Deli Meat and Subsequent Changes in US Regulatory Policy," *Clinical Infectious Diseases*, vol. 42, no. 1, August 7, 2005.

Gould, Hannah. "CDC Research Shows Outbreaks Linked to Imported Foods Increasing—Fish and Spices the Most Common," U.S. Centers for Disease Control and Prevention, Press Release, March 14, 2012.

"Government Guidelines for the Safety & Dangers of Plastic Containers (Including Baby Bottles and Microwavable Bowls)," *New Parents Network*, July 12, 2013.

Greiff, James. "What Was Arsenic Doing in Our Chicken, Anyway?" Bloomberg View, October 10, 2013.

Grillo, Christine. "The Science Is Clear: Antibiotic Resistance and Food Animal Production, Center for a Livable Future, March 13, 2012.

Grieve, Maud. "FDA: We Won't Ban BPA (for Now)," Botanical.com, March 31, 2012.

Gunther, Andrew. "Would You Like Extra Ractopamine With Your Pork, Sir?" *Huffington Post*, Huff Post Food," December 5, 2012.

Hariyanto, Joko. "Indonesia bans imports of U.S. beef," *Wall Street Journal*, April 28, 2012.

Hennessy, Maggie. "Food Industry Group Wants Permission to Label GMO Foods as 'Natural'," Food Navigator-USA, December 20, 2013.

Holt, Steve. "Finally: American Chickens Will No Longer Be Fed Arsenic," Take Part, October 2, 2013.

Hongyi, Wang. "Food Safety Tops Public's Concerns," *China Daily*, August 21, 2013.

———. "KFC supplier used excessive additives in chicken feed," *China Daily*, December, 21, 2012.

Hopkinson, Jenny. "Lawmakers Ask Obama to Keep '07 GMO Labeling Promise," Politico Pro, January 16, 2014.

Humane Society of the United States. "Undercover Investigation Documents Pig Abuse at Tyson Supplier," May 8, 2012.

———. "Rampant Animal Cruelty at California Slaughter Plant," January 30, 2008.

"Import Guidance." Seafish.org, August 2010.

"Indian Ban on Imports of U.S. Poultry Sparks WTO Dispute," International Centre for Trade and Sustainable Development, Bridges vol. 16, no. 9, March 7, 2012.

Institute for Natural Healing. "Processed Meats Too Dangerous for Human Consumption," updated, May 22, 2013, World Cancer Research Fund (WCRF).

"Investigation of an Outbreak: Pritzer, Fred, Foster Farms Plant Closed by USDA: Cockroaches Found, says Salmonella Lawyer," Food Poisoning Law Blog January 9, 2014.

Iwamoto, Martha, et al. "Epidemiology of Seafood-Associated Infections in the United States," *Clinical Microbiology Reviews*, American Society of Microbiology, April 2010.

Jackson, LeeAnne. "Overview of FDA's Food Defense Activities," U.S. Food and Drug Administration, Center for Food Safety and Applied Nutrition, January 26, 2012.

Jacobson, Michael F. "Letter to the Food Standards Australia & New Zealand," Quorn-brand imitation meat products, Center for Science in the Public Interest, September 22, 2010.

James, Susan Donaldson. "Kraft Agrees to Take Yellow Dye Out of Mac and Cheese," ABC News Good Morning America, October 31, 2013.

Jaslow, Ryan. "Taco Bell tied to 2011 salmonella outbreak that sickened 68," CBS News, February 2, 2012.

Kelber, Kara. "Consumers Union Applauds FDA Move to Ban BPA in Infant Formula Packaging," *Consumers Union*, July 11, 2013.

Kieler, Ashlee. "Potentially Harmful Chemicals Find Their Way into Our Food Thanks to 56-Year-Old FDA Rule," *Consumerist*, April 7, 2014.

———. "Study Finds Produce, Restaurants Most Likely To Give Consumers Foodborne Illnesses," *Consumerist*, April 8, 2014.

Kim, Susanna. "11 Food Ingredients Banned Outside the U.S. That We Eat," ABC News Good Morning America, June 26, 2013.

Kimbrell, Andrew. "Citizen Petition Before the United States Food and Drug Administration," Center for Food Safety, 2011.

Kirkpatrick, Kristin, "10 Things You Don't Know About Sugar (And What You Don't Know Could Hurt You)," HuffPost Healthy Living, July 30, 2013.

Kobylewski, Sarah, and Michael F. Jacobson. "CSPI Says Food Dyes Pose Rainbow of Risks—Cancer, Hyperactivity, Allergic Reactions," Center for Science in the Public Interest, June 29, 2010.

"Labeling Around the World," Just Label It, 2014. http://justlabelit.org/right-to-know/labeling-around-the-world/.

Landro, Laura. "Informed Patient: Danger in the Deli? Listeria Risks Go Beyond Cantaloupe," *Wall Street Journal* Health Blog, October 3, 2011.

Landsman, Jonathan. "The Unpalatable Truth: GMA Wants GMOs Kept Secret," Natural Health 365, May 19, 2014.

Larsen, Linda. "Raw Milk E coli Outbreak Sickens 12 in Missouri," *Food Poisoning Bulletin,* April 13, 2012.

"Letter to Sunland Inc. Concerning Suspension of Food Facility Registration; Notice of Opportunity for Hearing from U.S. Food and Drug Administration." November 26, 2012.

Levick, Richard. "Are GMO-Free Cheerios the First Domino?" *Forbes*, January 9, 2014.

Lewis, David L. et al. "Interactions of pathogens and irritant chemicals in land-applied sewage sludges (biosolids)." BMC Public Health, BioMedCentral, June 28, 2002.

Li, De-Ki, et al. "Urine Bisphenol-A Level in Relation to Obesity and Overweight in School-Age Children," PloS One, published by the U.S. National Library of Medicine, 2013.

Lohr, Steve. "Baby-food makers confront British contamination scare," *New York Times*, May 2, 1989.

Lupkin, Sydney. "Cyclospora Victim: 'I Found Myself in Tears a Lot of the Time'," Good Morning America, ABC-TV News, August 2, 2013.

Lyon, William. "Managing German Cockroaches," Entomology Fact Sheet, NHE-3, Cooperative Extension Service, University of Illinois, April 1996.

Maryland Environmental Health Network. "Maryland Children's Environmental Health Progress Report," January 17, 2013.

McGonigle-Martin, Mary. "Real Stories of the Dangers of Raw Milk," interview by U.S. Centers for Disease Control and Prevention, January 24, 2011.

Mead, Paul S. et al. "Food-Related Illness and Death in the United States," *Emerging Infectious Diseases*, vol. 5, no. 5, October 1999.

"Meeting of the National Center for Food Protection and Defense (NCFPD)." Chaska, Minnesota, June 28, 2007.

Melnick, Meredith. "Why Lovin' the McRib Isn't Heart Smart," *Time*, October 27, 2011.

Michigan Department of Agriculture and Rural Development. "Michigan Cottage Foods Information," 2014.

Milbank, Dana. "Budget cuts as back-door deregulation," *Washington Post*, April 2, 2012.

Moore, J. C., J. Spink, and M. Lipp. "Development and application of a database of food ingredient fraud and economically motivated adulteration from 1980 to 2010," U.S. Library of Medicine, National Institutes of Health, PubMed.com, 2013.

Nachman, Keeve. "Roxarsone, Inorganic Arsenic, and Other Arsenic Species in Chicken: A U.S.–Based Market Basket Sample," *Environmental Health Perspectives*, National Institutes of Health, 2010.

"Natural Astaxanthin—The Distinct Differences between Natural and Synthetic Astaxanthin. *Well Wise*, August 2000.

Natural Resources Defense Council. "Fix the FDA," 2014.

———. "Top 10 Reasons to Eat Grass-Fed Meat," August 19, 2011.

"Nearly Three-Quarters of Americans Looking to Government for More Food Safety Oversight," Harris Poll, New York, February 5, 2014.

Neil, Martha. "'Pink Slime' Beef Producers Sue ABC, Diane Sawyer, USDA Microbiologist and Others, Seek $1.2B," *ABA Journal*, September 13, 2012.

Neltner, Thomas G. et al. "Conflicts of Interest in Approvals of Additives to Food Determined to Be Generally Recognized as Safe Out of Balance," *Journal of the American Medical Association*, December 9, 2013.

North Texas Wellness Center. "10 American Foods that Are Banned Elsewhere," November 21, 2013.

Office of Environmental Health Hazard Assessment, State of California. "Chemical Listed Effective April 11, 2013 as Known to the State of California to Cause Reproductive Toxicity: Bisphenol A (BPA)," April 2013.

"Optimizing produce food safety is 'simply good business'—Price Waterhouse Cooper." *Bites*, Kansas State University, April 20, 2012.

Oregon Health Authority, Public Health Division, Office of Disease Prevention & Epidemiology, Acute and Communicable Disease Prevention. "Summary of the Foundation Farm Raw Milk-Associates E. Coli O157:H7 Outbreak," 2012.

Ostfield, Marc L. "Food Defense: The Vital Role of International Collaboration," remarks at the Biennial Meeting of the National Center for Food Protection and Defense (NCFPD), Chaska, Minnesota, June 8, 2007.

———. "Food Defense: International Collaboration in a Critical Area of Biodefense," Remarks to the European Institute: Transatlantic Dimensions of Biodefense Cooperation and Collaboration Event, Washington, DC, November 20, 2006.

"Outside the U.S." Fishwatch-U.S. Seafood Facts, September 6, 2013.

Painter, John A. et al. "Attribution of Foodborne Illnesses, Hospitalizations, and Deaths to Food Commodities by Using Outbreak Data, United States, 1998–2008," *Emerg Infect Dis* [Internet]. March 2013. http://dx.doi.org/10.3201/eid1903.111866, Centers for Disease Control and Prevention.

Paish, Matt. "Exclusive: World Food Safety Expert on Challenges in Delivery Food Safety in a Global Food Chain," AFN Thought on Food, Australian Food News, May 14, 2012.

Palleschi, Amanda. "Government Executive—USDA 'Playing Chicken with Food Safety,' Protesters Charge," Food Whistleblower, http://www.foodwhistleblower.org, April 2, 2012.

Palmer, Kim. "Raw milk sickens more than widely reported, study says," *USA Today*, December 11, 2013.

"Papaya Food Poisoning: CDC Update on Salmonella Agona Outbreak." CDC report, Food Poisoning Law Blog, July 27, 2011.

Pendrous, Rick. "Closer Scrutiny of U.S. Food Imports Promised," Food-Navigator-USA, March 2, 2011.

Pennybacker, Mindy, and P. W. McRandle. "Guide to Which Fish Are Safe to Eat," Organic Consumers Association, February 24, 2004.

Perl, Peter. "Poisoned Package," *Washington Post*, p. W08, January 16, 2000.

Pew Trusts. "Pew Initiative on Food and Biotechnology," April 2004.

Petro Chemistry—Europe. "Phenol & Acetone Sector Group," July 2014.

Pierson, David. "Costco unsure how cooked chicken was tainted in Salmonella outbreak," *Los Angeles Times*, October 14, 2013.

Pizzomo, Joe, Jr. "Genetically Modified Foods: Just Say No!" WebMD, Integrative Medicine and Wellness, November 20, 2007.

Polidoro, Ronnie. "Infographic: Americans Say Sugar is More Harmful Than Marijuana," NBC News/The Wall Street Journal Poll, March 13, 2014.

Powell, Doug. "58 sick; E. coli O157:H7 outbreak—it's over—linked to romaine lettuce," 7th International Conference for Food Safety and Quality, March 23, 2012. http://blog.usfoodsafety.com/2012/03/23/58-sick-e-coli-o157h7-outbreak-its-over-linked-to-romaine-lettuce/.

Pray, Leslie, and Ann Yaktine. "Managing Food Safety Practices from Farm to Table," National Academies Press, 2009.

"President's Food Safety Working Group." Fact Sheet, March 14, 2009. http://www.foodsafetyworkinggroup.gov/FSWG_Fact_Sheet.pdf.

Pritzer, Fred. "Foster Farms Plant Closed by USDA: Cockroaches Found, Says Salmonella Lawyer," Food Poisoning Law Blog, January 9, 2014.

Prue, Kalee. "Real Stories of the Dangers of Raw Milk," interview by U.S. Centers for Disease Control and Prevention, January 24, 2011.

"Public Health Dispatch: Outbreak of Listeriosis—Northeastern United States, 2002," *Mortality and Morbidity Report*, Centers for Disease Control and Prevention, October 25, 2002.

Quester, Brandon, and Tarryn Mento. "Salmonella Outbreak Traced to Cantaloupes in Guatemala," Center for Public Integrity, October 3, 2011.

"Rampant mislabeling of beef in Korea." Food Navigator-Asia, October 14, 2013.

"Recommendations for Improving Import Safety." Pew Health Group, Focus On: Food Import Safety, Food Safety Modernization Act, 2010.

Reinberg, Seven. "Better Safeguards Needed for Imported Food, Drugs: Report," *Health Day*, April 4, 2012.

Rettner, Rachael. "Will You Even Notice the Trans Fat Ban?" HuffPost Healthy Living, November 13, 2013.

Riggs, Julie. "Real Stories of the Dangers of Raw Milk," interview by U.S. Centers for Disease Control and Prevention, January 24, 2011.

Risher, Brittany. "Decoding the Deli Counter," *Women's Health*, January 30, 2014.

"Risk Assessment for Food Terrorism and Other Food Safety Concerns." CFSAN/Office of Regulations and Policy, Oregon State University, October 7, 2003

Roos, Robert. "GAO: USDA Took Shortcuts in Poultry Inspection Plan," University of Minnesota, Center for Infectious Disease Research and Policy, September 4, 2013.

Rowan, Karen. "Raw Milk Sickened Scores Despite Inspections," Live Science, May 1, 2013.

"Russia, U.S. to hold poultry talks in Moscow." *Ria Novosti*, January 19, 2010.

Ryan J. Foley. "U.S. Charges Egg Company, 2 Execs in 2010 Outbreak," ABC News, May 21, 2014.

"Salmonella Newport Outbreak Linked to Alfalfa Sprouts." PritzkerLaw, May 28, 2010.

"Salmonella Outbreak Is Traced." *New York Times*, April 17, 1985.

Schmidt, Charles W. "Organic Chicken Has Much Less Arsenic," Earth Open Source—Environmental Health Perspectives, 2012.

Schneider, Kate. "The ancient lost city of Shi Cheng lies deep underwater," news.com.au, February 20, 2014.

Schultz, Hank. "Advocate: People get ready, there's a non GMO train a comin'," Food Navigator-USA, August 8, 2013.

Schumer, Charles E. "Schumer Reveals: Toxic, Cancer-Causing Chemical That Subway Sandwich Chain Voluntarily Removed from Their Bread This Week Can Still Be Found in Scores of Other Fast Food Products; Calls on FDA to Ban Chemical in Food Nation-wide," website of Senator Charles E. Schumer, United States Senator for New York, February 10, 2014.

Shaw, Gina. "Despite Delays in Implementation of FSMA, the Food Industry Moves Forward," *Food Quality & Safety*, December/January 2013.

Silk, Benjamin J. et al. "Vital Signs: Listeria Illnesses, Deaths, and Outbreaks—United States, 2009-2011," *Morbidity and Mortality Weekly Report*, U.S. Centers for Disease Control and Prevention, June 4, 2013.

Simon, Michele. "A Budget Cut Only the Produce Industry Could Love," EatDrinkPolitics, February 28, 2012.

"Singapore." One World Nations Online, 2014.

Skae, Teya. "The Harmful Effects of Sugar and Choosing Healthy Alternatives," Natural News, February 21, 2008.

Snipes, Kate, and Carol Kamau. "Kenya Bans Genetically Modified Food Imports," Foreign Agricultural Service, U.S. Department of Agriculture, November 27, 2012.

Spinner, Jenni. "Doctors win $8m grant to look at BPA effects on babies," *Food Production Daily*, August 22, 2013.

Stevens, Shawn. "Seeds Implicated in Salmonella Sprout Outbreak Reportedly Imported From Italy," Food Safety Counsel—Gass Weber Mullins LLC, Food Safety Attorneys, May 6, 2009.

Strom, Stephanie. "F.D.A. Bans Three Arsenic Drugs Used in Poultry and Pig Feeds," *New York Times*, October 1, 2013.

"Sugar: How Much Are You Eating?" Pure Performance Physical Training, July 4, 2013.

"Prevention for a Healthier America—Investments in Disease Prevention Yield Significant Savings, Stronger Communities," article published in *Trust for America's Health*, at www.healthyamericans.org, July 2008.

"Sweet deal? Maybe not beware of honey sold in stores. It may not be honey." *Monroe News*, November 27, 2011.

"Taco Bell lettuce suspected in E. coli outbreak." CNN Money, December 13, 2006.

"Tentative Determination Regarding Partially Hydrogenated Oils; Request for Comments and for Scientific Data and Information," notice by the U.S. Food and Drug Administration on Federal Register, November 8, 2013.

Terracini, Benedetto, ed. *Toxic Oil Syndrome, Ten Years of Progress*, World Health Organization—Europe, 2004.

"Terrorism: Chemical Terrorism." Canadian Security Intelligence Service, Jewish Virtual Library, 1994.

Thompson, Dennis. "Stomach Bug Outbreak Cases Top 500," Health Day, *U.S. News and World Report*, August 8, 2013.

"Tomorrow Is Election Day." Elections, Eat Drink Vote, November 4, 2013.

U.S. Centers for Disease Control and Prevention. "Foodborne Illness Surveillance, Response, and Data Systems—CDC Estimates of Foodborne Illness in the United States," January 14, 2014.

———. "CDC Estimates of Foodborne Illness in the United States," January 8, 2014.

———. "Cyclosporiasis Outbreak Investigations—United States, 2013 (Final Update)," December 2013.

———. "Norovirus," October 30, 2013.

———. "Food Poisoning from Marine Toxins," Travelers' Health, August 1, 2013.

———. "*Infections from Some Foodborne Germs Increased, while Others Remained Unchanged in 2012*" April 18, 2013.

———. "Raw (Unpasteurized Milk)—Trying to Decide About Raw Milk?" February 25, 2013.

———. "Parasites—Toxoplasmosis (Toxoplasma infection)," January 10, 2013.

———. "Multistate Outbreak of Salmonella Braenderup Infections Associated with Mangoes (Final Update)," October 11, 2012.

———. "Multistate Outbreak of Listeriosis Linked to Whole Cantaloupes from Jensen Farms, Colorado," August 27, 2012.

———. "CDC Research Shows Outbreaks Linked to Imported Foods Increasing," March 14, 2012.

———. "CDC Study of Unexplained Dermopathy," January 25, 2012.

———. "Investigation Announcement: Multistate Outbreak of Salmonella Enteritidis Infections Linked to Restaurant Chain A," January 19, 2012.

———. "Investigation Announcement: Multistate Outbreak of E. coli O157:H7 Infections Linked to Romaine Lettuce," December 7, 2011.

———. "Pregnant or Older? Be Safe with Ready-to-Eat Meats," May 2011.

———. "2011 Estimates of Foodborne Illness in the United States," April 15, 2011.

———. "Multistate Outbreak of Human Salmonella Montevideo Infections (Final Update)," May 4, 2010.

———. "Multistate Outbreak of Salmonella Typhimurium Infections Linked to Peanut Butter, 2008–2009 (Final Update)," May 11, 2010.

———. "Salmonellosis," National Center for Emerging and Zoonotic Infectious Diseases, November 16, 2009.

————. "Investigation of an Outbreak of Salmonella Saintpaul Infections Linked to Raw Alfalfa Sprouts," May 8, 2009.

————. "Investigation of Outbreak of Infections Caused by Salmonella Saintpaul," August 1, 2008.

————. "Multistate Outbreak of Salmonella Litchfield Infections Linked to Cantaloupe (Final Update)," April 2, 2008.

U.S. Department of Agriculture. "Interagency Risk Assessment: Listeria Monocytogenes in Retail Delicatessens," Interagency Retail Listeria Monocytogenes Risk Assessment Workgroup, September 2013.

————. "MDP—Program Overview," last updated June 19, 2013.

U.S. Department of Agriculture, Food Safety and Inspection Service. "FSIS Comparative Risk Assessment for Listeria Monocytogenes in Ready-to-eat Meat and Poultry Deli Meats Report," May 2010.

U.S. Department of Health and Human Services, National Institute of Environmental Health Sciences, National Institutes of Health. "Bisphenol A (BPA)," May 22, 2014.

U.S. Department of Health and Human Services, National Toxicology Program. "Butylated Hydroxyanisole," in *Report on Carcinogens*, 12th edition (2011).

U.S. Department of the Interior, U.S. Fish and Wildlife Service, Division of Law. "Annual Report FY 2000."

U.S. Environmental Protection Agency. "Laws and Regulations," 2014. "Fish Consumption Advisories," June 9, 2014. http://water.epa.gov/scitech/swguidance/fishshellfish/fishadvisories/index.cfm.

U.S. Food and Drug Administration. "FDA News Release," July 12, 2013.

————. "Hazard Analysis & Critical Control Points (HACCP)," July 5, 2013.

————. "Dangers of Raw Milk: Unpasteurized Milk Can Pose a Serious Health Risk," June 17, 2013.

————. "Everything Added to Food in the United States (EAFUS)," April 23, 2013.

————. "Citizen Petition to Prohibit or Enjoin the Use of Antibiotics in the Production of Distillers Grains Sold as Animal Feed for Food-Producing Animals," March 15, 2013.

————. "Justification of Estimates for Appropriations Committees," 2013.

————. "FDA announces recall of cantaloupe by Chamberlain Farms of Owensville Indiana Farm's cantaloupe may be one source of contamination in multi-state outbreak of salmonellosis," News Release, August 22, 2012.

————. "Questions and Answers—Raw Milk," March 1, 2007, last update November 1, 2011.

————. "Melamine Pet Food Recall," October 7, 2009.

————. "T.M. Kovacevich International, Inc. Recalls Cantaloupe Because of Possible Health Risk," March 25, 2008.

————. "How U.S. FDA's GRAS Notification Program Works," December 2005/January 2006.

————. "Food Establishment Inspection Form," December 2003.

U.S. Government Accountability Office. "2012 Annual Report: Opportunities to Reduce Duplication, Overlap and Fragmentation, Achieve Savings, and Enhance Revenue, GAO-12-342SP," February 2012.

————. "FDA Should Strengthen Its Oversight of Food Ingredients Determined to Be Generally Recognized as Safe (GRAS)," March 5, 2010.

Valdes-Garcia, Yissel S. et al. "Growth performance and carcass characteristics in finishing feedlot heifers fed different levels of chromium-enriched live yeast or fed Zilpaterol Hydrochloride," *Cuban Journal of Agricultural Science*, vol. 45, no. 4, 2011.

Van, Jon. "'85 Salmonella outbreak largest ever, study says," *Chicago Tribune*, December 11, 1987.

Wagner, Sarah A. et al. "Adverse Effects of Zilpaterol Administration in Horses: Three Cases. Original Research," *Journal of Equine Veterinary Science,* vol. 28, no. 4, 2008.

Walla, Arjun. "Scientists Discover Bt Toxins Found in Monsanto Crops Damage Red Blood Cells," Collective-Evolution, May 11, 2013.

Wallinga, David. "Playing Chicken—Avoiding Arsenic in Your Meat," Institute for Agriculture and Trade Policy, Food and Health Program, April 2006.

Walsh, Rob. "Go Texan, Eat Local, Support Texas Cottage Food," Texas Eats, September 29, 2010.

Waltrip, Elizabeth A. "Inspections, Compliance, Enforcement, and Criminal Investigations," FDA letter, re: Sparboe Farms/Prairie Complex, November 16, 2011.

Wang, X.H. et al. "Assessment of the determination of azodicarbonamide and its decomposition product semicarbazide: investigation of variation in flour and flour products," *Journal of Agricultural and Food Chemistry*, Department of Food Services and Technology, Agricultural University of Hebei, People's Republic of China, published on Europe PubMed Central, 2011.

Warshaw, Hope et al. "Fat Replacers: Their Use in Foods and Role in Diabetes Medical Nutrition," *Diabetes Care*, vol. 19, no. 11, July 31, 1996.

Watson, Elaine. "Judge: 'There is a gaping hole in the current regulatory landscape for 'natural' claims and GMOs," Food Navigator—USA, June 18, 2013.

Weise, Elizabeth. "Mango recall follows 105 Salmonella cases in 16 states," *USA Today*, August 31, 2012.

Weiss, Bernard. "Synthetic Food Colors and Neurobehavioral Hazards: The View from Environmental Health Research," Environmental Health Perspectives, National Institutes of Health, U.S. Department of Health and Human Services, September 16, 2011.

Weitzman, Hal. "Four accused in US over tainted cheese," *Financial Times*, April 20, 2012. http://www.ft.com/cms/s/0/e2fcb6dc-8a4c-11e1-93c9-00144feab49a.html#axzz33QEVc2I.

"When Science Becomes Business When Business Runs Governments," America's Food Industry, http://multipletext.com/2013/11-1_Americas_food_industry.html.

"Where does the FDA stand on the use of Azodicarbonamide?" Examiner.com, February 26, 2014.

"Why Raw Sprouts May be the Riskiest Food in Your Grocery Store," HuffPost-Food, *Huffington Post*, June 11, 2011.

Wiedman, Martin. "Using Risk Assessment to design effective intervention—Case study: Listeria and deli meat," Department of Food Science, Cornell University College of Agriculture and Life Sciences, September 2013.

Wilce, Rebekah. "Under Pressure, Whole Foods Agrees to Stop Selling Produce Grown in Sewage Sludge," PR Watch, January 16, 2014.

William, Scott. "Wake Up America and Read the Label Next Time," Scribd.com, 2013.

Winslow, C.-E. A. "An Outbreak of Tonsillitis or Septic Sore Throat in Eastern Massachusetts and Its Relation to an Infected Milk Supply," *Journal of Infectious Diseases*, vol. 10, no. 1, January 1912.

Yang, Quanhe et al. "Added sugar intake and cardiovascular diseases mortality among U.S. adults," National Institutes of Health, PubMed.gov, U.S. National Library of Medicine, April 2014.

Zemser, Rachel. "No You Can't Sell Cottage Cheese Our of your Cottage Food Operation," FoodProductDesign.com, April 30, 2013.

Zerbe, Leah. "FDA: We Won't Ban BPA (For Now)," *Rodale News*, March 30, 2012.

Index

About the Author

Charles M. Duncan, an award winning TV investigative reporter, began researching and writing about food safety issues in 1970, producing and researching articles on lax food inspections in restaurants and contaminated kitchens in Wichita, Kansas, and the Dallas-Fort Worth area. His focus on potentially deadly pathogens from health violations in restaurants, food production plants, commissaries, schools, hotels, nursing homes, and hospitals resulted in major improvements in food safety.

Duncan's 18-month embedding in a top secret U.S. Customs and Bureau of Alcohol, Tobacco, Firearms and Explosives investigation of an illegal British arms dealer gave the public an inside view of a federal sting operation. His reporting became the first and only such journalistic milestone. He also attended and secretly videotaped a meeting between Cuban Mafia members and Florida state lawmen posing as part of a South Florida mob.

Duncan's vast journalistic experiences include his probes of security and health violations at Kelly Air Force Base in San Antonio, investigations into religious cults, the hazardous chemical industry, and many others. ABC's *World News Tonight* and *Good Morning America* aired many of his productions. Other media reporting on Duncan's works include *TIME, Newsweek, The Sunday Times* (of London), *Texas Monthly, D Magazine, Dallas Observer*, and numerous newspapers across the United States.

Duncan currently continues his scrutiny and probing of major food safety issues and dangers around the world.